BLUEBIRDS

Everyone was doing their part, now it was up to me. From a dead start I had to use all the acceleration to reach the boat's top speed by the time I went into the measured kilometre. Then, once out of it, I needed a controlled reduction of speed at the far end of the run. For a new record to be recognised, even unofficially, it has to show an increase of 2 per cent over the existing one, so relentlessly I forced my speed up and up. After a run towards Michael and Dean at 127 mph I was aware that Michael was looking at me less happily than he had done earlier. He could see that I was getting very excited. I was enjoying it so much that I couldn't wait for them to say, 'Right, return run,' and I'd be away. The record breaking bug had taken over and I was beginning to take it all fairly nonchalantly. I wouldn't say that I was becoming disrespectful but I was savouring every moment of the experience. Then after an upward run of 127 mph, I did the return one at 118 mph, and by the time I pulled alongside Roger and Terry on the jetty the timekeepers had said over the radio that the average of the two had given me a new Women's World Water Speed Record of 122.85 mph.

Me? I just sat there and stared and stared into the distance. The physical and nervous exertion had drained me. I, who just minutes before had been high with confidence and determination, felt like a wet rag. I'd set up a new record, and it was done. I had travelled faster over water than any woman before me. So what? Already it was something which happened to me in the past. Somehow, I felt my father was not far away, and I knew what had driven him and my grandfather on and on.

About the Authors

Michael Meech is a broadcaster, who first met Gina Campbell when he interviewed her for the BBC World Service programme, Outlook, in 1984. As a reporter and presenter he takes part in Current Affairs, Sport and Music programmes. He is also a popular speaker on Foyels list of lectures.

Gina Campbell is the daughter of Donald Campbell, one of the greatest speed boat racers of our time, who was tragically killed when he was trying to go just *too* fast on Coniston Water in 1967. She is the grand-daughter of Sir Malcolm Campbell, the flamboyant romantic amateur who broke all land and water speed records in the 1930s. Gina herself is the fastest woman in the world on water and she hopes to remain so.

Bluebirds
The Story of the Campbell Dynasty

Gina Campbell with
Michael Meech

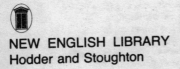

NEW ENGLISH LIBRARY
Hodder and Stoughton

In memory of Donald, my father, and the three ladies in his life and mine – Daphne, Dorothy and Tonia.

Copyright © 1988 by Gina Campbell and Michael Meech

First published in Great Britain in 1988 by Sidgwick & Jackson Limited

First New English Library paperback edition 1989

British Library C.I.P.
Campbell, Gina
  Bluebirds : the story of the Campbell Dynasty.
  1. Racing cars. Speed records. Campbell (Family)   2. Racing motorboats. Campbell (Family)
  I. Title   II. Meech, Michael
  796.7'2

ISBN 0-450-51111-X

This book is sold subject to the condition that it shall not, by way of trade or otherwise, be lent, re-sold, hired out or otherwise circulated without the publisher's prior consent in any form of binding or cover other than that in which it is published and without a similar condition including this condition being imposed on the subsequent purchaser.

No part of this publication may be reproduced or transmitted in any form or by any means, electronically or mechanically, including photocopying, recording or any information storage or retrieval system, without either the prior permission in writing from the publisher or a licence, permitting restricted copying. In the United Kingdom such licences are issued by the Copyright Licensing Agency, 33–34 Alfred Place, London WC1E 7DP.

Printed and bound in Great Britain for Hodder and Stoughton Paperbacks, a division of Hodder and Stoughton Ltd., Mill Road, Dunton Green, Sevenoaks, Kent TN13 2YA. (Editorial Office: 47 Bedford Square, London, WC1B 3DP) by Cox and Wyman Ltd., Cardiff Road, Reading. Typeset by Hewer Text Composition Services, Edinburgh.

PREFACE

The name of Bluebird passed from one car to another, from track racing to world speed records, from land to water, from father to son. In the passage of time, as world record succeeded world record, each became one more milestone of human progress, a single word in a book of human endeavour, a book perhaps, without an end. A book in which every man has something to write of his struggles, successes and failures on his ascent of the mountain of progress. But each can only go so far since the mountain has no summit, for it leads to the stars. It has to be climbed, for mankind cannot regress; he may pause momentarily, but there is no going back on the path of life.

In bygone days disease took a toll which progressing science is giving us the means to overcome; it is also giving us the means to totally destroy. With our faith in God, right has always triumphed over might. In the words of Thomas Edison, 'What the mind of man conceived, man's character can control.' Life is an eternal challenge, a variant on Maeterlinck's theme that the Bluebird of happiness is by the side of each and every one of us, always within reach yet, if pursued to catch and possess, is beyond our grasp. Man is given only two real sources of happiness – a happy marriage which means a happy home, and the satisfaction of a job well done. If this is true, the theme and the variant are synonymous and inseparable, for one without the other is like a dish without flavour, a day without sunshine.

DONALD CAMPBELL

1

'She's tramping . . . the water's not good . . . I can't see much . . . I'm going . . . I'm on my back . . . I've gone.' With those words over his radio my father came to the end of his career in record breaking, and to the end of his life. His boat, *Bluebird*, reared up and then crashed through the surface of Coniston Water on 4 January 1967, and remains there as an underwater memorial. His body was never found.

Seventeen years later, speeding across the lake at the National Water Sports Centre at Nottingham, I felt myself going up and up – and over backwards. 'My God,' I shouted over the intercom, 'holy shit . . . I'm coming up to join you, Dad.' I, too, was heading skyward at 160 miles an hour, and there was nothing I could do about it.

Record breaking is a bug which gets into your system. When my father decided to take over where Grandfather had left off he was warned, 'Once you start this thing, you're not going to be able to quit.' The addiction had taken me over completely that afternoon in October 1984, when I had just set a new Women's World Water Speed Record. True, like all women's records in my sport, it was unofficial – but only in the sense that the governing body, the Union Internationale Motornautique, behave as though speed on water is the prerogative of men. Official or not, I was just faintly disappointed that I had to be content with 122.85 when I had hoped to match my grandfather's first record on water of 126.33 at Lake Maggiore, on the border of

Switzerland and Italy, almost fifty years before.

But my support team were ecstatic. 'We've broken the record and we can do better still,' was their attitude. That compulsion within me to go faster and faster, combined with my desire to equal or exceed my grandfather's achievement, made me a willing partner to their enthusiasm for another run.

For a record to be established the timekeepers take the average speed for two runs made within twenty minutes of each other, in opposite directions over a measured kilometre. There was no time to lose. If only I could do another good run within the time limit I could push the record up by quite a lot.

In the heat of the moment it was decided to remove the boat's air spoiler. I knew well enough that this was a fairly important piece of equipment, but I never doubted the advice I was being given. It was a higher record we were after, and getting rid of the down-thrust which the air spoiler created would increase our potential speed.

Perhaps there were lingering doubts in my subconscious for I know that I said to Roger Jenkins, who owned the boat, 'Do I do anything different?' I'll never forget his reply. 'Eyes down and welly it. Eyes down and welly it,' he said twice, in what I took to be a somewhat uncompromising tone.

No one could have begun an attempt on a world record with more cryptic instructions! I already knew that Holme Pierpoint, the lake at the National Watersports Centre at Nottingham, was only two kilometres long. This meant that I had just 500 metres to get up to my top speed, and then I had to not lift my foot off at all until I passed the 1500 metre sign. After that, 500 metres remained in which to slow down. Bringing a powerboat to a standstill from such a high speed is tricky. You have to ease up very gently. If the nose comes down into the water too suddenly a front-first, end-over-end somersault can begin, with disastrous consequences.

The driving felt little different to me. In a few hours

I had come to love and enjoy my borrowed boat. There was something almost feminine about her appearance, yet as I pulled away from the jetty behind me there was the thrust of a rocket. Already I was the fastest woman on water and I was confident that within minutes I would have raised my speed still further.

To me, there is something strange about the fact that Holme Pierpoint is stocked with freshwater fish. There was I, determined to make my small contribution to history, and around the bank were countless fishermen more concerned that my wake would disturb the surface than they were interested in watching a minor milestone in speed on water. But I have to remember that fishing is as much a watersport as powerboating.

Regardless, my business was to set a new world record. Behind me was the powerful roar of the engine, ahead the nose lifted above the surface, and I knew we were trailing out that white plume of spray which had been a Campbell hallmark for three generations now. It was exciting – and humbling. The boat was as stable as before and I had no sense that we were going any faster than we had done on our previous runs that day.

Gradually at first and then more violently, I began to take off. Instead of looking at the horizon I was seeing the sky. My distant point of focus had been across the water to the shore of the lake, but without warning everything was blue and flecked with fleecy clouds. I remember trying to look down, and thinking, 'God, don't look there, girl.' I was going up and up, and something was pressing on my nose. It was the air pressure on my visor. I knew Bluebird was doing a backward somersault and, in terror, it was then I shouted, 'My God . . . holy shit . . . I'm coming up to join you, Dad.'

I was being thrown over backwards in the air, and by the time I realised it I knew I was beyond the point of no return. I have a loathing of being splashed with water but in those hundredths of seconds – no, thousandths

3

of seconds – my mind said, 'This time, Gina, you won't mind getting wet, because if you feel wet you'll know you're all right.' And there, upside down in the boat, about to be thrown out at any moment, eighty feet above the lake, I said, 'Please God, let me feel wet – let me get wet – because if I'm wet, I'll know I'm OK.' Even in the split second while it was all happening I realised the similarities with the accident in which my father had been killed and, to be honest, I was convinced I would be killed too.

The next thing I was aware of was a sort of glug, glug, glug; that strange sound which you get as you rise to the surface after jumping into the deep end of a swimming pool. I was wet, very wet, but I was alive. I was even thankful for the coldness of the water, as it had brought me round from the momentary blackout I must have suffered as I was flung out of the boat, as I had experienced no feeling of flying through the air.

Breaking the surface I was amazed to see how far I was from the boat, or what remained of it. The largest piece was just sinking, and there were bits and pieces of debris everywhere. The marine ply had splintered and now looked like soggy cardboard. In a strangely childish way I felt that I was to blame. I was so upset and remember thinking, 'Oh God, I've broken it.' Immediately I knew that this was the end of record breaking for the foreseeable future. That beautiful boat was not there any more. Part of the machine which had inspired and carried my hopes was now floating wreckage, the rest a hulk embedding itself at the bottom of a man-made lake.

It was a friend's interest in offshore powerboat racing rather than any deliberate plan of my own which had started me off. He talked and I listened; he drove and I watched. Then I realised that I was wasting my time and decided to have a go myself. It was even more of an accident that within a year of beginning I decided to challenge for the Women's World Water Speed Record.

My boyfriend, Michael Standring, and I decided to do some offshore racing as a pair for pleasure, but without much conviction that trophies or championships would follow. But there is something in my family which means that you only take part in this purposeless way once. From then on, you're there to win. With our interest now directed more positively, but with precious little evidence of our ability, by the beginning of the 1984 season we had the sponsorship of Agfa-Gevaert, the British branch of the Belgian and German reprographic company. In March that year *Agfa Bluebird 1* was launched. The press were invited to St Katharine's Dock, at London's Tower Bridge, to see her and there was an overwhelming response. It was, in a way, a tribute to my father and grandfather, and also a response to the name Bluebird which in their days had been synonymous with record breaking on land and water.

Suddenly the enormity of what we'd embarked upon came home to Michael and me. With the names Campbell and Bluebird everyone was going to expect more of us than we might be able to deliver! It was too late now and we would have to live up to it as best we could.

Amanda Slayton, Agfa's public relations lady, unwittingly committed us further by the way she wrote the press pack for the launch. She listed the full powerboating calendar for the season – races at Portsmouth, Southampton, Brighton, Fowey, Brixham, Torquay and so on – and then the final item in the calendar, as though to be taken for granted, Windermere Records Week.

Amanda knew what she was doing. No sooner were the formalities over than a pressman was asking me which record I was going for. I was flummoxed. Until that moment the idea of going for a record had never entered my head. 'Oh . . . oh . . . which record am I going for?' I addressed the question to myself, hoping he'd think I was being guarded about my intentions. Sensing my uncertainty, another press representative jumped in. 'You will be going to Windermere Records Week, will you?' 'Of course,' I replied, mustering as much charm as my embarrassment would permit. 'In this boat?' they asked. 'Yes, in what else?' I said. At that moment I knew that we had let ourselves down. *Agfa Bluebird 1* was a splendid boat for offshore racing but was by no means a record breaking boat. Our absence of plans had been exposed. I hope that in the intervening years I have become less inept at dealing with press enquiries. The pseudo-friendly approach of journalists – use of my Christian name, and reference to my father – can be beguiling. In the end, they will write what makes the best headline. In spite of this, I have come to regard the newspapers, radio and television as allies. My rule is always be prepared to listen to their questions or be photographed, and always have something to say which they can report, but when I am unsure of myself or my plans – as I was at the launch – I admit it, and never allow myself to be drawn into saying what I had decided to keep private.

The line of enquiry was pursued over lunch by Ross Nott and Fiona Brothers. Both write for boating magazines, but at different times have held the Women's World Water Speed Record. Very quickly I learned not to be drawn into conversations with the press which could hold little or no advantage for me. I suspect they saw me as an unworthy pretender to their throne, so I was very cautious.

All the way home my mind was whirling around thinking about attempting the women's record. 'It could be something really exciting,' I thought. Michael had heard the general questioning, but did not know that Ross and Fiona had cornered me later. Like me, he felt that there was a possibility – and we would both enjoy the challenge. But there were a million and one obstacles, not least getting a suitable boat and meeting the expense.

A day or two later we had a phone call which offered

a solution to my problem. Michael took it and, after a series of yesses interspersed with pauses, called me to speak to a Roger Jenkins. My reaction was to ask, 'Who the hell's Roger Jenkins?' Michael said he thought he was once a World Inshore Circuit racing driver. In a very broad Welsh accent Mr Jenkins confirmed what Michael had said, and went on, 'I understand that you want to do a world record.' Again I was guarded. He was so direct in his approach but there was warmth and enthusiasm in his manner.

Before I could mutter more than a syllable or so, he went on, 'You won't do it in that old tub you've got, as you well know, but I've got the boat for you.' He'd got it all worked out in his mind already, and without a pause, he continued, 'I can teach you to drive it and with my expertise, my schooling, and everything else, you'll be the fastest lady in the world on water. And you'll do it in two days.'

With what I can best describe as a chuckle, I suppose I conveyed both pleasure and uncertainty. 'Well, do you want to do it or not?' he came back to me. Sounding, though not feeling, indignant that anyone should need to ask, I said, 'I'm game.'

'OK then,' he said, 'don't breathe a word to anybody – keep it absolutely dead quiet to yourself, and we'll set something up.'

Looking back now I realise how audacious I was to go along with the idea of attempting the record. Michael and I were newcomers to the powerboat racing fraternity, and my experience as a driver was minimal. I'm not sure whether I was a hero or a fool – or both – but the risks involved in a novice, as I was then, attempting such a feat were monumental. Had they known what I was planning, I'm sure that more qualified drivers would have advised me against tackling the record so early in my racing career. But they did not know, and I was swept along by Roger's enthusiasm and my own dedication to the family's record breaking heritage.

I never clapped eyes on Roger Jenkins for another six months. We had one or two telephone conversations but didn't meet until I was at Ipex – the big International Printing Exhibition – at the National Exhibition Centre at Birmingham. *Bluebird* was on display there for Agfa. Alongside they had a large hospitality unit where they entertained favoured customers and friends, and I was doing my PR bit signing autographs and patting small boys – and larger ones – on the head.

Roger Jenkins was coming to meet me and the Agfa management for lunch. As soon as he arrived I liked him. He's small, very open and very brash. All of us were transfixed by the Rolex watch on his wrist: it was the biggest any of us had ever seen, and it was covered in diamonds. We were all sitting there thinking, 'Twenty, twenty-five grand, do you reckon?' He had a big BMW outside and he'd arrived with stickers saying 'Campbell's Bluebird World Record Team' all over it – talk about putting the carriage before the horse.

Over lunch Roger hammered out a deal with Bob Dickenson, who was the managing director of Agfa and to whom I owe a lot, and Tony Burton, who runs their Reprographic Divison. We were going to lease Roger's boat, paint it in the Agfa colours, also with the name Bluebird, and have Roger with his team and equipment to set up my attempt on the Women's World Water Speed Record.

For the second time in six months we called the press together to see another *Bluebird*. On this occasion we were beside the Serpentine, in Hyde Park, in London. I, too, was seeing her for the first time and was so proud. This beautiful boat was going to make this little lady somewhat more worthy of the Campbell heritage.

Our plan was to take the boat to Windermere to make my attempt during Records Week, but before that I needed to familiarise myself with the craft which was very different from anything I had driven before. I needed to do this almost in secret, and two days

8

later we met Roger with the boat in Nottingham, at the National Watersports Centre. As she was unloaded from the truck I knew I'd fallen in love with her. She looked so beautiful, I wanted to touch and caress her. More than any other boat I have known this *Bluebird* was a real 'she'.

I'd not slept the night before as I was so nervous. It was not fear of what I was about to do which kept me awake but the sheer exhilaration of knowing that I was being backed to make this attempt on a world record. To some extent I had bluffed my way into this situation. For months I'd been bragging to myself and my friends about what I could do given the chance. This was the day on which I could prove it.

Just in case the weather was nasty at Windermere and we were not able to run the boat, Roger had taken the precaution of inviting the official timekeepers from the Royal Yachting Association to come to Nottingham. Having them in attendance was a ploy my father often used when he did not want publicly to say that he was going for a record.

Roger got into the boat, and went off like the clappers. He was obviously doing nearly a hundred but still had time to take his hands off the wheel and give us a wave. For me it was ''Scuse me, where's the ladies?' time!

As I put on my helmet and lifejacket I noted that a special boat with a stretcher and a doctor on board was standing by, and on the bank there was an ambulance. My instructions were to go up and down the lake again and again until I felt at home with this lovely craft. As I climbed aboard Roger explained how to start it: switch on fuel pumps, hold heater like choke, count 1, 2, 3, and then bump push the starter. It was like a horse kicking you up the jacksey when it fired as it was immediately in gear.

Gently I went backward and forward up and down the lake, venturing from forty miles an hour up to sixty and then seventy. At seventy I got into what seemed like a violent wheel wobble except that the boat appeared to be swinging sideways as well as up and down. 'Wow, there's something terribly wrong here,' I thought, and gingerly crept back to the jetty. 'Ah, that's the porpoise,' said Roger, 'you've just got to have confidence at that stage to keep your foot down hard and drive through it. Believe me, it'll be all right.'

Fifteen minutes before, I had never been in this boat. She weighed 1000 lb and had a 550 hp engine which enabled her to leap from zero to 100 mph in about 3½ seconds. And now, if my attempt on the record was to be realistic at all, I had to take her to twice the speed at which it seemed the whole thing was going to shatter into pieces. 'Off you go,' Roger said. 'Gradually build up to seventy and then go through the porpoise this time.' There seemed to me to be no point in fooling about at lower speeds now that I knew what I had to do, so I kicked her into life again, put my foot down and within two seconds she was porpoising. Four seconds later we were through it. I felt as cocky as hell, I really did! I kept slowing down and then building up the speed again, knowing how the boat would react. I had mastered it.

Back at the jetty Roger was both pleased and cross with me. He called me a 'little monkey' and said, 'I told you to settle down and wait until the wash had subsided before you tried to beat the porpoise.' But it was a step in the right direction, and I know he was glad really. A huge grin spread across the face of his engineer – Big Terry – and he said in his Birmingham accent, 'I can see you've done a hundred 'cos the flies have stuck to your visor, and they don't do that under a hundred.'

At such a moment how anyone could think about stopping for lunch, I don't know, but this splendid team I had around me suddenly decided to go off and eat cheese and raw onion sandwiches. I mean, I love cheese and onion sandwiches, but I was keyed up and ready to go and their concern to eat made me livid. I might have had just a cup of coffee – I don't really remember – but nothing more. My adrenalin was pumping hard as I knew they were all expecting a lot of me. A BBC camera crew were there to shoot some footage for a documentary they were making about me, so any mistake was going to be well chronicled, and, you know how it is, if you know that you must not make a mistake you have a horrible feeling that you'll make one. Michael was a great help at this stage. He kept telling me how well I was doing, and how proud he was of me. He was very supportive with sound advice and pleas to be careful. Roger, meanwhile, was bubbling over with excitement. 'We'll have a record by two o'clock,' he told the camera team, 'and then we'll be on the piss!'

With lunch disposed of, and all of them stinking of raw onions, I got back into the boat and could see at once that they meant business. Perhaps my anger at them for wanting to stop for lunch had been misdirected. I had been tense and had forgotten for the moment that anything I could achieve depended on these guys who were sharing the strain with me, and without their specialist knowledge and experience I could do nothing.

They began to weigh out and measure the fuel. In a boat in which the power to weight ratio was so finely balanced, the amount put into the tank was an important consideration. They decided on five gallons, which seemed to me to be quite a lot when you remember that fully dressed I weigh only 8 stone 2 lb. While this was going on, the timekeepers took their places in the little huts provided for them at the 500 and 1500 metre marks. Roger and Terry stayed at the start, while Michael and Roger's son, Dean, went to the far end of the lake, to provide a base for me there.

Everyone was doing their part, now it was up to me. From a dead start I had to use all the acceleration to reach the boat's top speed by the time I went into the measured kilometre. Then, once out of it, I needed a controlled reduction of speed at the far end of the run. For a new record to be recognised, even unofficially, it has to show an increase of 2 per cent over the existing one, so relentlessly I forced my speed up and up. After a run towards Michael and Dean at 127 mph I was aware that Michael was looking at me less happily than he had done earlier. He could see that I was getting very excited. I was enjoying it so much that I couldn't wait for them to say, 'Right, return run,' and I'd be away. The record breaking bug had taken over and I was beginning to take it all fairly nonchalantly. I wouldn't say that I was becoming disrespectful but I was savouring every moment of the experience. Then, after an upward run of 127 mph, I did the return one at 118 mph, and by the time I pulled alongside Roger and Terry on the jetty the timekeepers had said over the radio that the average of the two had given me a new Women's World Water Speed Record of 122.85 mph.

Roger just threw himself about. He flipped himself over backwards and lay – wearing his designer gear and gold watch – in all the seagull muck. He got up, kissed his radio, embraced me, put his arms round the shoulders of the men and shook their hands, and went into a sort of impromptu victory dance. The Welsh have always been more demonstrative than we phlegmatic English!

Me? I just sat there and stared and stared into the distance. The physical and nervous exertion had drained me. I, who just minutes before had been high with confidence and determination, felt like a wet rag. I'd set up a new record, and it was done. I had travelled faster over water than any woman before me. So what? Already it was something which happened to me in the past. Somehow, I felt my father was not far away, and I knew what had driven him and my grandfather on and on.

In a strange and contradictory way, I was intensely proud of what I had done, yet for the first time I sensed, as they must have done, that the build-up to the record attempt is more exhilarating than being a record holder. I had crossed one threshold but another lay waiting to be crossed.

Being in this frame of mind I was bound to respond to Roger's and Terry's suggestion that we should try to increase the speed still further. And there was the competitive quality within me which wanted to do as well as my grandfather had done when he first held the World Water Speed Record. Together, diminutive Roger and big Tel had all that I needed in terms of skill, experience and judgement, so I never doubted that we should and could do better.

If a further run was to be valid, it had to be done within twenty minutes. We had little time to spare. With hindsight, I can see that when we removed the air spoiler we should have realigned the engine in relation to the boat. It never crossed my mind, and obviously neither Roger nor Terry thought of it either. I really believed in them – and still do. Roger had set records himself and knew that they never come easily or without risk. I have to admit that at this stage Michael was becoming slightly disenchanted with Roger, perhaps because he was less directly involved in the action and so much closer to me in personal terms. He went rather quiet and told me afterwards that he felt a bit of a coward because at that moment he knew we were taking a chance with my life.

Neither our hopes nor Michael's fears were realised in the event. We lost the boat, but I was safe. Quite quickly the rescue boat was alongside me. Very carefully the men lifted me from the water as they were not sure how badly I was injured. In fact my chin was grazed and my nose was painful as it had been flattened by the visor, but my main concern was that I was drenched from head to toe. They urged me to sit down but I just wanted to remain standing, let the water run out of my racing suit and dry off.

My first thought was Mr Woppit. 'Have you got my teddy?' I asked. One of the divers got him for me even before they put a tow rope on what remained of the boat. Mr Woppit is an important figure in my family's record breaking tradition. He is a teddy bear, about eight inches tall, who went almost everywhere with my father. He was the last thing to go on board in all of Dad's record attempts and the first thing off afterwards. Although no trace was ever found of my father after the accident in which he was killed on Coniston Water, Mr Woppit floated to the surface and he was passed on to me some years afterwards by Tonia, who was Dad's wife at the time of his death. When I started racing I took Mr Woppit on every trip and that afternoon at Nottingham he had been strapped to the steering column of the boat. He is, I think, one of my most treasured possessions and I was more glad than I can say to have him back.

On our way back to the jetty I tried to make light of what had happened with silly remarks about women drivers and the like as I didn't want them to think I was a sissy or a wimp who was going to cry. It was a nervous reaction more than anything else. As they helped me from the boat onto the jetty one of the rescuers who was more cheeky than the other said, 'Cor, Gina, it's good to see you're still smiling.' Only then did I realise that the seat of my racing suit and my panties had been torn to shreds and he was looking at the cheeks of my bum and not the cheeks of my face!

I needed the hugs I received as I was by then so cold – so very, very cold – and I didn't have anything to keep me warm. To Roger I was pathetically apologetic, like a child who'd just broken a friend's toy, as I had smashed his beautiful boat which I had loved so much.

Michael reacted very quickly and took me off for a hot bath but, frustration of frustrations, we simply could not find the women's shower room. Realising that shock could be setting in he pushed me into the men's and said that he would keep guard outside. At that stage I think

14

he was more shocked than I was. I'd not been in the shower above a minute or two when there was a loud hammering on the door. Now Michael is not the kind of person who loses his cool very quickly, but I heard his voice raised and soon he was effing and blinding for all he was worth which is quite out of character. I discovered afterwards that a man who had just finished a game of squash wanted a shower too and, though Michael explained the gravity of the situation and our predicament, he did not give a damn. Michael was so protective and I thought it was nice that he stood up for me.

Of course, I had to see the doctor who was present and, along with everyone else, I think he expected me to be in a state of mental shock. I assured him I was fine and his very thorough examination confirmed that there was no sign of serious damage.

Happily I got in a quick phone call to my mother in Devon before the world's media arrived. I knew how worried she would be if what had happened was mentioned on the radio before I could reassure her that all was well. But I was only just in time. From nowhere, it seemed, within minutes they descended on me: newspapers, television cameras, radio, the lot. I suspect one of those apparently uninterested fishermen on the bank had tipped them off as soon as I had flipped over.

The end of my precious *Bluebird* – really it was Roger's, of course – was sadder still. When the team got the wrecked boat up on the ramp and onto the trailer Roger could see that there was a lot of damage to the £25,000 engine. The boat had been completely submerged with only the ends of the two hulls sticking out above the surface of the lake. Rapidly they started stripping the engine down but there was an awful lot of fuel around. There must have been a spark – and woomph, the whole thing went up in flames.

By this stage, as I said, Michael was somewhat disenchanted with Roger and, to him, there seemed to be

15

poetic justice in his precious snap-on tools – the best that money could buy – being pushed into the water when his crew attempted to put out the flames. It was ironical to see the divers afterwards using magnets in an attempt to locate those prized socket sets.

I didn't feel the impact of the accident until a few weeks later when I was shown some photographs of an Italian driver having exactly the same accident as I did. As he was thrown into the backward somersault, I could see the moment when his neck broke. I went cold. I could not take my eyes off the picture. My stomach suddenly fell out of me. I thought, my God, that could have been me. It was so close, and he was killed. It was horrible. He was upside down in the air with his heels nearly touching the back of his head.

I've often been asked whether I would do it again. If I do it will be in part to prove to myself that I have the guts to face what I know to be a hazardous pursuit, and the test will come only when someone says, 'There's a boat – get into it and have a go.' In 1984 the Women's Record was described by the authorities as 'unofficial' as at that time there was no distinct recognised category for women within the sport. That's changed now and the temptation to go for an officially recognised record is always there. It was the Countess of Arran – who's still racing at the age of sixty-nine – who claimed the initial record for a woman. She was the first woman to do more than 100 mph on water and since then Ross Nott and Fiona Brothers have sustained a tradition of which I am proud to have become a part. There is no sense in which I feel that I have emulated my father. I feel that I've been on a glorified ego trip, but one with a purpose. I had to exorcise my past. I was told time after time that my father and grandfather were such great men; England, Europe, the whole world admired their daring, the King and Queen recognised their heroic qualities. Yet there was I, an abysmally pathetic child who had not achieved anything. The day I broke the record I liberated myself from this burden and felt that I had lived up to the Campbell inheritance. I had been where they had been and come back with that sense of pride and awareness of human frailty which were characteristic of them.

Everybody around me says that achieving the Women's World Water Speed Record has changed me. Michael says that a new self-confidence was evident at once and I think, without being cocky, that that is true. It is not the self-confidence born of feeling that I'm superior but of knowing what I have managed to do. 'Hell, I'm Donald Campbell's daughter,' I say to myself. 'If anyone else wants to come and improve on what I've done, let them come and show me how.' In the days when I was show-jumping and I'd done everything I could in a competition and someone came along and said, 'You should have pulled him up here, kicked him there, or pulled him off then,' I'd say, 'I'm getting off. You show me how well you can do it.' They never did. I'm ready to learn from people who have done what I am trying to do more successfully than I have, and to follow their guidance, but I have no time for the armchair experts who have never soiled their hands, been bruised and sore, or got their buttocks wet. When I knew that the Women's World Water Speed Record was mine I felt a kind of confidence was justified and I still do. If there's another woman who's prepared to do what I did, and better it, then she should go ahead. That is probably the challenge I need. But four years later there has not been one.

2

If you want to understand me and my story then you have to know something of the feelings I have for my father. In many ways they are irrational as relationships of love and admiration often are. Other people have said that he did not treat me fairly, and even that he would have preferred me to be a boy so that there was a greater chance that I would grow up to share his enthusiasm for things mechanical. For my part, I don't see him through rose-coloured spectacles though it would be easy to do so in view of the way his life ended. None of us is perfect, and neither was Donald Campbell, but for me he is the most complete man I have ever known or am ever likely to know. I'm biased, of course I am, and why shouldn't I be? He was my father! He had charm and good looks, he was courageous and fun-loving, his integrity was beyond question and he had a single-mindedness which made him a winner when again and again circumstances conspired to defeat him.

The first time I recollect seeing my father he was in his study at Abbots, our house between Reigate and Dorking, in Surrey. He was about five feet eight inches tall, about the height of all the men of the Campbell family for several generations back. He looked healthy and, though there was nothing to indicate it when first I remember him, I know he was quite strong. His dark hair was slightly receding which, with his unlined face, gave him an immediate appearance of openness. What we called the study was more of a den, and it gave hints of the boyhood which he had

18

only reluctantly left behind. There were the drawings and bits of equipment which go along with being a born engineer, and around the walls he had pictures of Neville Duke, who was a long established friend, and the aircraft in which Duke had won the World Air Speed Record. At one stage he installed a public address and radio relay system throughout the whole house and I can remember jumping out of my skin on more than one occasion when I was in my bedroom alone and his voice came out of the loudspeaker asking, 'Georgina, what are you doing? Could you come to the study, please?' If there was something on the radio which he thought everyone should hear, without warning the programme would be fed from his study to all the rooms in the house. This kind of technical mischief gave him a lot of pleasure. He enjoyed building the equipment and he had fun using it whether for a serious purpose or to take someone unawares. I don't remember, and perhaps I never knew, whether he was able to listen in to conversations in other rooms from the study, but I would not be surprised if he could!

Never did I see my father unshaven. He was a meticulously clean man – particularly about his fingernails which is very surprising when you think how much grease and grime he came into contact with. Whenever he went to London, or to a business meeting, he would wear the very best worsted wool suit with a tailored silk shirt with Bluebird or his initials monogrammed on the breast.

He was once nominated one of the best dressed men of the year and when this was announced I remember his secretary, Rosemary Pielow, having hysterics as she was used to seeing him at home in a jumper frayed at both cuffs and a hemline stretched out of all recognition, a sports shirt with a threadbare collar, sagging flannel trousers and a pair of dirty old yachting shoes. 'Here comes one of the best dressed men of the nation,' she would say, 'and look at him now!'

There was one notable occasion when he abandoned his immaculate personal presentation and that was during the time he was married to Tonia and the three of us were on holiday in the South of France. We were walking along La Croisette, a very smart street in Cannes, and Tonia and I chose to walk a few steps behind him because he insisted on wearing some ex-army shorts which covered his knees, leaving his hairy white legs exposed like a typical English tourist. Around us were lots of trendy young Frenchmen in nicely fitting designer shorts. When we pointed out how out of place he looked all he said was, 'They're comfortable.' Making him laugh was always rewarding and I know that at one stage I picked up one of those silly schoolgirl riddles at school and so I asked him, 'Why does Victor Sylvester always wear baggy pants?' The answer was, 'So that he's got more ballroom.'

My father was born at Povey Cross, his parents' home in Surrey, in March 1921. His mother was my grandfather's second wife. There seems almost to have been a conspiracy of silence about his first marriage. Throughout my life I have asked questions about it but no one has been able – or willing – to tell me anything about it. The only thing I have managed to glean is that she was 'a lady of some presence' and some of those who knew them thought it was monstrous that Grandfather had been so unpleasant that she felt it necessary to leave him and bring their marriage to an end. It is strange that in a family that is mostly so well documented her memory has been almost completely eradicated.

Daddy had a sister, my Aunty Jean, who was two-and-a-half years younger than he was, and with whom, according to Dad, he 'played, fought and found trouble'. A couple of months after my father was born, Leo Villa joined Grandfather as his racing mechanic and he proved to be a wonderful confidant and companion to Dad, and later to me.

From the outset Father was surrounded by cars, oil,

the sound of tools on metal and talk of racing or record breaking. My grandfather, Malcolm, was a very determined man from all accounts, and most of all so about his driving. I did not know him, but most of the people who did conveyed to me the impression of someone who was very austere, yet it is obvious that Dad had a closeness to him which few others seem to have achieved. As children, he and Jean would hide while Grandfather was bathing and shaving in the morning. When he came out of his dressing room he would pretend not to be able to find them, and when he did there would be a real rough and tumble with gales of laughter from them all.

This was the setting for Father's first boxing lessons. Grandfather had some small boxing gloves made for Dad and from a kneeling position would show him how to land a punch, or evade one an opponent was trying to deliver. One day Jean pleaded to be allowed to join in, and Grandfather agreed but said that, to be fair, Dad had to have one hand tied behind him. She was more effective as a boxer than either had expected and really hurt Dad with one of her punches. In anger he hit her very hard on the nose. In tears she fled, bleeding profusely, her interest in boxing at an end.

Povey Cross, where they lived, reflected my grandparents' well-to-do lifestyle. A long, curving drive led from the road to the house which was surrounded by a maze of paths on which Daddy and Jean used to stage races in their pedal cars and later on their bicycles. There were kennels, a tennis court, a sunken garden and pond, an orchard and four acres of fields as well as the superbly equipped workshop in the outbuildings. The staff included a governess, from whose attention my father delighted to escape, the butler, a cook, a housemaid, and a couple of gardeners.

My father's misshapen right ear was a relic of those days. Carlos, one of the Alsatians which Grandfather kept, was a very friendly dog but one day while standing with his forepaws on Dad's shoulders he snapped at a fly and took a slice out of his ear. Dad found the iodine which was applied by his mother more painful than the bite!

To keep such an extensive garden spick and span frequent bonfires were necessary, and Grandfather had developed a particular pleasure in getting a good blaze going. It was an enjoyment which Donald and Jean quickly came to share and they would set light to patches of dry grass in remote parts of the estate and then argue about whose turn it was to be the fire brigade and stamp it out. It all went happily until they lit some grass near one of the haystacks, and in next to no time flames were leaping sixty feet into the air and yellow smoke billowing across the field. Dad dashed into the house and found a small hand fire extinguisher, but the real fire brigade had to be called to put out the blaze. Fortunately no one ever told Grandfather how one of his haystacks came to catch on fire.

Some of Father's misdemeanours began with good intentions. Finding some creosote which the gardeners had left over after treating a fence, Daddy felt that the stone surrounds of the goldfish pond would be improved with a coat of it. He didn't realise how much of the creosote went into the water, but Grandfather did the following morning when many of the goldfish were dead. His nose twitched as it always did when he was annoyed, Dad told me, and he repaid Father for his trouble with a riding switch.

One of Dad's more interesting problems as he was growing up was Malcolm's total commitment to anything he did. Daddy remembered being given an electric train set one year at Christmas, but within weeks Grandfather had taken it over, extended its track, increased its rolling stock, and forbidden Dad to play with it unless he was present. The pretext for this was that within a few hours of receiving it my father's technical curiosity prompted him to begin taking the engine apart. In his supervisory role, Grandfather enjoyed it so much that he had the train set moved to a large disused barn where he extended it. All this Father could tolerate, but when it was sold to one of the big London shops and set up as part of their toy department he was both sorry and annoyed.

Malcolm Campbell wanted to be the master of whatever he did, and he would even compete with his children to prove that he was better at something than they were. A case in point was when Dad and Jean began to learn to play golf. It had never been Malcolm's game but in a very short time not only was he playing but having a nine-hole course laid in the grounds of Povey Cross.

Father also told me of Grandfather's fascination with buried treasure. He had been on several expeditions abroad in the hope of striking it rich but he never did. Then it occurred to him that the people who had built Povey Cross would have needed to keep what was precious to them somewhere. He decided that they would have buried their valuables in the garden, and Dad spent one exhausting weekend as foreman's mate while Grandfather led a team of diggers in excavating a large part of the garden. Their only success came when during the following week Grandfather borrowed an electric sensor which indicated that there was metal under one part of the lawn. Carefully the digging began and, after some time, was rewarded – with a rusty tin chamber pot which had lain there for years!

Grandfather became so intrigued with the sensor that he wanted to give it a further test, so he asked one of the staff to bury quite a lot of my grandmother's jewellery at various points in the grounds, without telling him where. Next day he set about finding it with the sensor, but was only partially successful. Some of it was never found. How he explained this to the insurance company – or to my grandmother – I do not know.

Schooldays began for Daddy at Horsham and continued at St Peter's in Seaford. From there he went on to Uppingham, the public school which Grandfather had attended. He found sport and practical studies like carpentry and photography more to his liking than academic work, and distinguished himself by remaining in the same form for three successive years at one stage. For all that, I am sure he was happy there, judging by the way he spoke of those years and the fact that I remember him having a photograph of himself in school uniform up in his study. The uniform consisted of a black tailcoat, pinstripe trousers, a shirt with a stiff collar and a black tie. I find it difficult to imagine any boy, least of all my father in his youth, caged in such clothes, going bird's nesting or riding a horse bareback, but he assured me that he did. In 1985 I had the honour of going to Uppingham School to unveil a plaque in West Deyne House, commemorating the fact that both Father and Grandfather had attended the school and been members of that house. Both also left their mark on the school in the form of initials carved on a beam in the dormitory which they used.

By the time he went to Uppingham Father could already drive. Grandfather had bought an old-style Morris Oxford for a few pounds, which Leo Villa converted into a pick-up truck. It was useful for hauling light loads, but quite soon he and Jean, under Leo's guidance, were able to drive it over the fields near their home. There is no need to ask who they pretended to be in the driving games which followed.

At that stage Dad and Jean used to spend part of most summer holidays at Bracklesham Bay, in Sussex, with a Mr and Mrs Burt, who were lifelong friends of the family. They had a very ancient motor bike, which eventually they gave to Daddy. He was thrilled. Although he was only twelve, he immediately went off to the nearest florists on it, to buy some flowers for Mrs Burt as a thank you present. When he came out of the shop he could not get the bike started. After persistent efforts it fired very suddenly and Dad, the bunch of flowers and the motorcycle were all thrown into a nearby ditch, where the old-fashioned open flywheel gouged out quite a deep wound in his leg. Undaunted, he had hours of pleasure out of this antique machine, until he drove it into a pond, after which, in his words, 'It never went quite so well.'

The mishap with the motor bike was only one of many which dogged him in his early years. It was as though fate, which undermined so many of his later record breaking attempts, was even then working against him. When he was old enough to ride legally he had two other motorcycle accidents after one of which he was unconscious for two days, and on both occasions took weeks to recover. When he went to Switzerland with Grandfather on a record attempt, he developed cramp while swimming in Lake Geneva and nearly drowned. A bad bout of rheumatic fever kept him in bed for several months early in his childhood, but he was at least rewarded with a summer in Cannes recuperating. This may well explain the constant back pain which he had to put up with, while the rheumatic fever was later to frustrate his ambition to fly with the RAF.

Only my father could sustain severed nerves in an elbow working in an office. His first job was as a very junior office boy with Alexander Howden & Co., who were insurance brokers in London. The managing director was an acquaintance of Grandfather's and Dad remembered being introduced to him on his first morning. Mr Tweddles' attempt to put the young Campbell at ease had the opposite effect. 'If he's got as good a nose for business as his father,' he told the manager of the motor department, to which Dad was allocated, 'he'll be a great credit to us.' At that moment Daddy was not sure that he had, nor was he sure that he wanted to be in the insurance business. It was in one of his less busy moments that he slipped while fooling around with one of his contemporaries, and went through a plate glass window, injuring his right elbow quite seriously.

As Father was by then earning a wage, Grandfather stopped his allowance. With an income of £2.50 a week, Dad's life had some strange contrasts. He was woken each morning by the footman, who laid out his clothes for him, and the butler served him a traditional breakfast alone in the vast dining room. The chauffeur brought his battered Morris Cowley to the door, and off he went to Tadworth station, where he took a third class ticket to London. With his limited means, a sandwich was all he could afford for lunch.

During the two weeks that Dad had to stay at home from work following his elbow injury, Grandfather left for the United States where he was to meet Henry Ford. By this time Grandfather was a director of Ford in Britain, and his mission was to tell the great man that a design feature of a new car the company was building was unsuitable for British conditions. None of the other directors apparently dared to challenge the great car builder's judgement, but Malcolm was sent and convinced Mr Ford of the wisdom of his suggestion.

If you take a nostalgic view of the thirties, which many people do, it is hard to imagine that car theft and damage to vehicles was a problem to the police in Surrey in those days. It had, in fact, taken on such proportions that the local police formed a flying squad of special constables on motorcycles to deal with the incidents. The work was part-time and voluntary, and suited Father down to the ground. Although he may have chosen to ignore the law himself occasionally, he was basically a law-abiding, patriotic citizen. What's more, there was the opportunity to ride a motorcycle to some purpose, and pit his wits and skill against those of the offenders. As a bonus it involved wearing a uniform consisting of peaked cap, jacket and knee breeches in blue, and black gaiters. I'm not sure how many felons he deterred or apprehended, but he became the chief constable's special messenger and it gave him his first taste of public service.

While serving as a member of this flying squad, Dad

became friends with Brian Hulme, who was later to marry his sister, Jean. Brian's first visit to Headley Grove was memorable. Brian was an attractive man, with a love of speed and sense of devilment which appealed to Daddy. On the afternoon of his visit, he drove up looking immaculate in his special constable's uniform, with his motor bike specially cleaned for the occasion. My father had hidden himself in the undergrowth next to the drive and just as Brian was passing fired a long burst with an automatic rifle into the tree above his head. What Brian said no one remembers, and perhaps that's just as well, but at least he knew that a family who could indulge in such an initiation rite was somewhat out of the ordinary.

My grandfather's obsession with speed had made him a renowned racing driver long before Dad was born, and he held the World Land Speed Record for the first time when Daddy was just over a year old. The whole of my father's childhood was set against a quest for speed. His first real involvement was just before the war in 1939, when Grandfather launched the latest in the line of *Bluebird* boats, and he invited my father to perform the naming ceremony. Dad recalled the moment when he smashed the bottle of champagne and said, very proudly, 'I name this craft *Bluebird*. May God bless her, her pilot and all who work with her.'

The trip to Coniston for the launch was memorable, because, as far as I can gather, it was the first time that Grandfather allowed Dad to drive when he was present. On the way they stopped for lunch and, noticing that Grandfather appeared rather tired after all the work he'd been doing to get the new *Bluebird* ready, Dad asked if he should take over. The old man agreed and, after receiving more than adequate paternal instructions about his driving, Dad set off. After doing a few miles at fifty, as instructed, Dad sensed that Malcolm was beginning to doze, and before long his head had fallen to one side and he was sound asleep. The fifty became sixty, the sixty became seventy . . . they were in the Lake District much sooner than they had planned. 'You kept to the fifty, did you, son?' asked Grandfather, looking at his watch. 'Of course, Father,' Dad replied. 'Bloody liar,' said Malcolm wryly.

My grandfather foresaw the onset of the Second World War, and wrote a couple of booklets and pleaded in speeches for the armed forces to be made ready. When the then Prime Minister, Neville Chamberlain, returned from his historic conference with Hitler in Munich, holding aloft a piece of paper which both had signed, and claiming that it guaranteed 'peace in our time', Grandfather was incensed by the superficiality of it all. So convinced was he that war was about to begin, that instead of attempting a water speed record in Switzerland in 1939, he went to Coniston, rather than risk being stranded in Europe if hostilities started.

On a more domestic note, Grandfather was anxious that if there were an invasion the Germans should not get his very fine collection of family silver. Some of it he had inherited, much he and my grandmother had bought, but there was also a large collection of trophies. With war imminent he packed it all into several large metal boxes and had it buried on a small island a short distance from the shore of a lake, at Tilgate House, in Sussex, which he owned.

The story does not end there, though. When the threat of invasion had passed he went with some of his men to recover the silver, but it seems that someone must have had an eye on him when it was buried, and had beaten him to it. More than half of it has never been found.

Grandfather's concern about the war meant that Daddy was ready to serve King and country, and he set his heart on being a fighter pilot. The war was not many days old when he went to the recruiting office and volunteered for service in the Royal Air Force, hoping to fly Spitfires or Hurricanes. The medical examination followed within a few weeks but presented no problems,

28

though he confessed afterwards that with a panel of medical officers looking at him he felt as though the words rheumatic fever were written all over him. He was told that as soon as possible he would be called for aircrew selection, the recruiting officer adding, in that strange way which officialdom has when faced with a dedicated enthusiast, 'Don't make a nuisance of yourself by writing or telephoning this centre.'

It seemed like an eternity before he was sent for to go to the RAF station at Cardington, near Bedford, where his flying potential would be assessed. He had been so preoccupied with the thought that they would not accept him if his history of rheumatic fever was detected that it came as a shock on the day before the selection board when one of his fellow recruits said how important maths is to a pilot or navigator. That evening Donald sat in a hut at Cardington trying to catch up on all the maths which he had forgotten or never learned.

Maths was important in the interview, but he managed all right. With current affairs he bluffed and guessed well enough to get by. When the doctor presented him with a list of illnesses, including rheumatic fever, and asked if he had suffered from any of them, he looked firmly ahead and said, 'No, Sir.' He was accepted as a trainee pilot with the extremely humble rank of A/C 2, and given the RAF number 964147.

Knowing that he was soon to join 'the few' seems to have released within Dad the swashbuckling spirit which characterised the men who fought and won the Battle of Britain. It had always been there in Malcolm Campbell, yet the fact that it was so much in evidence in him appears to have inhibited it in Donald until then. But that day at Cardington he had a purpose in his own right, he was free, he was a man.

Like so many of us at that stage, he decided to prove his maturity by testing his sexual prowess. Whether he was a virgin until that time I do not know, but in the manuscript of an unpublished book which he wrote he

29

tells how he spent a somewhat dramatic night at the Kit-Kat Hotel in Jermyn Street, in London's West End. 'Life was for living,' he wrote. 'There was no point in planning for tomorrow, because no one knew if there was going to be one. Life was for living today and I was living it.' In the middle of the night there was an air raid, and at two in the morning he was making love to a very beautiful girl to the hellish background of bombs falling and guns blasting. The noise was unbelievable and the walls were visibly shaking. Suddenly there was a deafening crash, he was struck a blow on the back of his head and stars of all colours flashed in front of his eyes. He was next aware of being on the floor knowing that the hotel must have suffered a direct hit and would be engulfed in fire at any moment. He knew this was the end and prepared to face the inevitable with equanimity.

Slowly, he realised that apart from a sore head he was very much alive. Very gingerly he picked himself up from the floor. Beside him the lovely girl was still out cold. He could then see what had happened; the expansive double bed had collapsed, the solid wooden headboard breaking away from the rest and falling on the two of them. 'It was a terrible anti-climax,' he says, but whether this refers to the air raid or their lovemaking is not clear.

It must have been on the same visit to London that Daddy met Malcolm and went with him to a private exhibition of paintings at Marlborough House, the home of Queen Mary. A few of the visitors were selected to be presented to Her Majesty, who was a very imposing lady. As a very raw recruit, still feeling very uncomfortable in his RAF uniform, Aircraftsman Campbell was one of those chosen. As he moved forward rather nervously, he heard himself being announced as 'Admiral Sir Gordon Campbell'. Queen Mary looked at him rather quizzically and said dryly, 'I think there must be some mistake.'

Father's hopes of flying were short-lived. He thrived

on the prospect until he was called up, but then, within no more than a day or two, he was told at the Medical Centre that an electro-cardiogram had revealed that he had suffered from rheumatic fever in childhood. He pleaded to be allowed to stay in the flying branch but there was no way in which anyone could send him forward for aircrew training with such a history. To stay in the Air Force in some other capacity would, as he saw things, mean that he had started by being beaten and that he could not accept. He went home to civvy street in a mood of disappointment, depression and despair, such as he never knew at any other time in his life.

For the early part of the war he worked for a firm which had invented a secret device to be used in the defence of airfields. While the Battle of Britain, from which he had been excluded, went on in the skies above southeast England, he was on the ground installing and checking equipment which protected Fighter Command. It was as good a second best as he could have hoped for.

Later he moved to a firm which, under Grandfather's and Leo's guidance, had converted many Bedford trucks into armoured cars for the Home Guard in 1940. By the time Father joined them they were producing aircraft spares and other ancillary equipment for the forces.

The war, which at times had seemed phoney or distant or both, was by then much more real and immediate. London and southern England were being bombed regularly. My father particularly recalled the terror created by the flying bombs and V2s which were used towards the end of the war. At the factory he worked off the tension in energetic games of rugby, which put the lie to the idea that he had a suspect heart.

Shortly after the war ended, Grandfather sold Headley Grove to the Maharaja of Baroda and acquired Sax Rohmer's old house on the outskirts of Reigate. Sax Rohmer was the author of mystery novels featuring Fu Manchu. Whether it was because of this or not Father never said, but the house – though in a lovely position – had an intriguing atmosphere.

Not long after they moved in a family party was being arranged and, at the last moment, my grandmother suggested inviting an old school friend of Jean's, Daphne Harvey. Daphne accepted, and the result was a very happy evening throughout which my father had eyes only for her. The following Sunday Donald went to see Daphne and met her mother and stepfather at their beautiful home at Lock, near Partridge Green in Sussex. He was very impressed. The house stood in 2000 acres, and there were stables and a number of beautiful hunters. Daphne was an accomplished horsewoman and, although only twenty-one, was joint master of the local hunt. They saw more and more of each other, and soon enough were head over heels in love.

For some reason, which I cannot understand, neither set of parents approved of the friendship. Somewhat reluctantly, they agreed to them becoming engaged, but with the proviso that they wait a year before getting married. Before the engagement became official Mr and Mrs Harvey had second thoughts, and one day when Dad and Daphne met in London she had to tell him that she had been forbidden ever to see him again.

Both of them were strong characters and could not take such a prohibition lightly. They sat in silence in Dad's car, parked by the edge of the Serpentine, for some time. Quite suddenly their eyes met, and simultaneously each said to the other, 'Let's go and get married.' Their next stop was Caxton Hall Registry Office, where they applied for a special licence to marry.

Then they had to face the music. Daphne's family were at Claridges, prior to leaving for a holiday on which she was supposed to be going. When they told her parents the news, a storm broke. Andrew Harvey – a big, imposing Scot – in a booming voice, which echoed through the foyer of the hotel, told Father exactly what sort of blackguard he thought he was. His adjectives were of the most colourful. In seconds the place was in an uproar with guests, managers and porters looking on as the altercation moved towards the front entrance. With typical humour my father said that it was all he could do to stop himself standing to attention in military style, to show what he thought of Mr Harvey's attitude.

In the street outside, Andrew Harvey turned his wrath on Daphne, while her mother pleaded with Daddy. A policeman came round the corner and Mr Harvey shouted to him, 'This heinous fellow is stealing my little girl!' 'Oh no he's not,' Dad put in, and produced their birth certificates. Politely but firmly and perhaps with a twinkle in his eye, the constable said that this was a civil matter and not within his jurisdiction.

Daphne and Father jumped into his car, but, to their horror, Mr Harvey stood immediately in front of the bonnet, so that they could not move an inch. Quick-thinking as ever, Dad reversed away, then plunged the car into first and was off down the street. With hearts still pounding they drove down to the Campbells' family home in Surrey, where Daphne was to take shelter until the wedding.

All Daphne's clothes, possessions, and her car – an MG which she treasured – were still at Lock. They decided that the only way to get them was to drive there that same evening. While they were bundling all the things from Daphne's bedroom into the back seat of Dad's car, one of the staff phoned her father at Claridges to let him know what was happening. His response was to say that in no circumstances were they to be allowed to leave, and that he would be home within the hour.

Dad and Daphne went to the garage to collect Daphne's MG only to find that it had been immobilised. The chauffeur who had phoned Mr Harvey had acted swiftly and removed the rotor-arm from the distributor. By sheer good fortune, the family Rover was parked in the next garage and the rotor-arm from that fitted the MG. As they pushed the MG out into the moonlight and started the engine, the chauffeur appeared from his upstairs flat, pleading with them not to go. 'Oh dear God, I shall lose my job,' he wept. 'I shall be sacked. Miss Daphne, do you realise what you're doing to me?' 'Go to hell,' said Dad. 'You should have realised that when you were interfering,' and they were away.

Again on the following Monday morning when the wedding was to take place, someone let Daphne's parents know the time and place of the event. Donald had wanted his parents to be present, but with crisp, military precision and vocabulary, Grandfather declined so that Grandmother, too, had to stay away. It must have been a strange occasion with one set of parents refusing to be present, and the other rushing to get there in time with the sole intention of stopping the wedding happening at all. Caxton Hall saw some remarkable weddings as it was chosen by many of the great and famous as the place to exchange their vows, but Dad and Daphne's wedding must rank among the most unusual.

Dad remembered the chief registrar that morning in 1945 as combining the formal and the sensitive, and his room was brightly decorated with lovely flowers. In the absence of family or friends, Dad had to go out into the street and ask a couple of complete strangers to come in and act as official witnesses.

Daphne's stepfather arrived just as the ceremony was to begin. With emotion and anger he implored Daphne to relent and, eventually, the registrar had to ask him to leave as other couples were waiting. Mr Harvey left in considerable distress, Dad said, and although he was sad to see someone so upset at such a solemn moment, he said he had to fight to control his sense of the ridiculous, as the occasion seemed like a shotgun wedding in reverse.

Outside in Caxton Street, as Daphne and Donald left, Mr Harvey was still ranting and raving, by now including threats to kill my father in his repertoire of abuse. The previous week's scene at Claridges was repeated. After

Daphne and Donald had had their wedding breakfast alone, as they drove off a now near demented Mr Harvey clung to the car, shouting for his little girl to get out and come home. The indignity of it all – outside Claridges!

Though Daphne had been in the army, she came from a very strait-laced family. Donald's pugilistic, devil take the hindmost attitude to life – and particularly to those who opposed him – appealed to her. It was a rebellion against her parents' conventional expectations, and she enjoyed it.

Marrying Donald meant that my mother had to try to relate to the rest of the family as well, and this she did not find easy. Grandfather was a showman but had a very hard nature. At times he was tough and quite unkind, and never once does she remember him putting his arm round her, or giving her a kiss. He was very proud of his title and she always called him Sir Malcolm, rather than Father, Dad or Pa. Most of all she found his attitude to the man she loved hard to bear. She recalls how dictatorial he was with both Donald and Jean, and would say to Donald, 'You're never going to be as good as me. We aren't built the same way – you haven't got the guts that I have.'

For all that, he was quite kind to my mother. She remembers him as a small, wiry man with particularly strong wrists and hands. He always wanted the workshops to be tidy, and was a perfectionist in his appearance. He wore beautifully tailored suits and handmade shirts, and always had the right clothing for anything he was doing. He was willing to spend money on himself, his cars and his boats, but he was mean towards other people. Daphne, rather mischievously, wonders whether she was welcomed into the family because she had some money of her own, and was not likely to be a liability to the Campbells!

Headley Grove was an imposing house with large rooms and high ceilings, and it was lavishly carpeted everywhere. Many of the rooms were curtained with white velvet, and there were white cushions on the chairs and settees which looked very impressive, but were not at all practical. It is true that by the time my mother knew them, Malcolm and Dolly Campbell were on the point of getting their divorce, but there was no feeling that the house was a home which people lived in and enjoyed. It was more an exhibition of affluence. Their friends were few, and most of them contacts made through the world of motor sport.

With such a large house a considerable staff was needed. As well as the manservants, there was a housekeeper, a cook, and an array of kitchenmaids and chambermaids as well as the chauffeur and the gardeners. It was a relic of Victorian England which had outlived its day, and all the staff knew they had a master who kept them in their place with the lowest of low wages, and rigid discipline. My mother sees Leo Villa in her memory as the one who stood out as the kingpin of the whole Campbell operation. He worked himself almost to death and when anything went wrong had to take a lot of stick. In the end, Grandfather left him a house and a car.

Daphne found my grandmother – Dorothy Campbell, or Dolly – a puzzling person, though in many ways she was very fond of her. She had been described as the most beautiful woman in Surrey, and it was a beauty that remained until she was into her nineties and living in a nursing home. She had been born in China where her father had been an official of the British Government, and was largely brought up by a Chinese nurse, who taught both her and her brother to speak a Chinese dialect. That background seems to have given Grandmother a mask-like expression, so that no one ever knew quite what she was thinking. She was always beautifully dressed and wore expensive jewellery, but she was greedy for good things, and became slightly jealous of anything out of the ordinary my mother had. Dolly could not bear Mother to wear a Russian sable stole, which her mother had given her. She borrowed it on several occasions and eventually asked Daphne to give it to her.

In a sense, Dolly had the same problem as all Donald's wives had later on. The men they loved, and who in their way loved them, had a fascination with speed, and their women had to take second place. Dolly went along with Grandfather's passion for racing for a long time, but gradually found it more and more unbearable, and began to create for herself an independent life.

Daphne says that the only piece of domestic furnishing she and Daddy possessed for their first home was an ashtray, so they were fortunate to find a house in Kingswood, in Surrey, which belonged to a couple who were moving abroad and wished to dispose of chairs, tables, carpets, curtains, cutlery, glass, kitchen utensils and garden tools as well as the house itself.

I am told that even my birth was surrounded by the same tempestuous aura which attended any event in the family Campbell. Daphne was a smart and attractive woman, and had done her best to conceal her pregnancy for as long as possible. Maybe that is why I have always been a compact person! Apparently I was overdue and my mother was uncomfortable, so she suggested to Daddy that he should take her for a drive late one evening to ease the tension she was beginning to feel. She told me that, as usual, he drove like hell. When they went straight over a solid heap of tarmac she hit her head on the roof of the car and was left wondering what sort of child she was going to produce.

Very early next morning, Mother had the first signs that my birth was imminent and Dad rushed her by car to London, where she had been booked into the private wing of Westminster Hospital. They were horrified to discover that there had been a mistake in the dates and that no private room was available. Instead they were put into a rather ordinary labour room, and my father was told by a young nurse that he could leave and that the hospital would be in touch with him later in the day. 'No bloody fear,' he said, 'if my wife has to be in this inadequate ward, I'll stay with her.' The matron was called, and heated words between her and my mother followed, which concluded with Father deciding that the best place for me to be born was back at home in Kingswood.

No preparations had been made for a delivery at home, so the sudden change of plan created another crisis. My grandmother remembered a doctor who had been very good when she was young, and got on the phone to him. My mother – by then well advanced in her labour – remembers him coming into her bedroom, stroking his chin and saying, 'Ah, yes,' and then disappearing. In time he returned, accompanied by the district nurse, equipped only with a half-empty bottle of ether and an inadequate supply of cotton wool. With the help of a nurse whose midwifery was at best rudimentary, and a doctor who was short-sighted and rather deaf, I made my entry into the world.

While all this was going on indoors, Mother tells me that Dad decided that it was the day to cut down a tree which had been taking quite a lot of light from the house. With a friend and a bottle of whisky, he set about the task, taking a breather from time to time to dash into the house to ask, with boyish enthusiasm, 'Have we got anything yet?' and later, 'What have we got?' By late afternoon I had arrived and Dad's first sight of me was as I lay on the bed with three dogs around me, and a host of grown-ups who all knew they should be doing something but were not quite sure what. One of the happiest aspects of the occasion was that Mother's old nanny moved in to care for both of us during my first few weeks, and provided a reassuring presence for her.

Mrs Harvey, my maternal grandmother, never really forgave Mother for marrying, but my grandfather on that side of the family, who had been so irate at the time of the wedding, was much kinder and came to see us and gave my parents some financial help. I claim no credit for it but, so the story goes, unconsciously I won the heart of Malcolm Campbell, and both he and Dolly took a great interest in their infant granddaughter.

My own first recollection of life is a naughty one. As a very little girl, when I used my potty I was not allowed to get off until an adult was handy to deal with the necessary details of hygiene. One day, when I had spent a penny, in spite of calling out for help nobody came to assist me so I stood up and poured the contents over my head – I was walloped for it!

3

Turbulent and unorthodox though my family may have been I would not change it for any other. We are unable to escape from our past and mostly I would not want to. The present is always full of frantic activity, and dreams which may never come to fruition. We would prefer at any time to make a wrong decision rather than stagnate through inactivity. More than most, we know that tomorrow is not promised to anyone, yet we plan as though it were already ours. I always hope that I can balance temerity of spirit and respect for nature and science as they did. So far I no more than live in their shadows.

My father's achievements – in his time more than now, perhaps – were measured against those of my grandfather. Malcolm Campbell was a British hero and known worldwide for his record breaking, and to an adoring public it seemed impossible when he died that there was another Campbell waiting in the wings to take up the role.

I think I know how Daddy must have felt; I have lived with the tension of being proud to be Donald Campbell's daughter yet longing for people to accept me for what I am myself.

My grandfather died on New Year's Eve 1948. I have no recollection of him but have always been fascinated by the mark which he left on the family and the wider world. From things my father said, I am left with admiration for him as a pioneer of speed on land and water, but it is a cold, remote feeling. He was an arrogant, self-opinionated man who would have merited the term male chauvinist pig had it been in fashion when he was alive. The only place for women, in his view, was in bed. Even Leo Villa, who worked with him as an engineer, said of him after he failed to be the first man to exceed 200 mph on land, 'He had always been difficult; now he became impossible.'

In fairness to Grandfather, I have to say that if he had been a milk-and-water London businessman, he would never have pushed world speed records beyond what seemed possible or reasonable, or thrilled the hearts of so many people in the way he did. In anyone who has the guts to push out the boundaries of human experience the sod factor has to be high.

Sadly, and yet amusingly, his pig-headed qualities also had their appeal. By the last few weeks of his life his brief third marriage had been dissolved and his sight was failing. He suffered his second stroke, and his doctor told him that on no account was he to leave his bedroom for a month. But no advice was as good as his own ideas for Malcolm, and within two days he was out on the road in one of his cars.

It had been Grandfather's custom to lay a wreath on my great-grandparents' grave at Chislehurst, in Kent, each year at Christmas. On his way home he had to ask Leo to drive. A day or two later he insisted on taking the car into Reigate where Reg Whiteman, his former butler, was to do his Christmas shopping. Again Leo was with them and recalled afterwards how, while Reg Whiteman was at the shops, Grandfather slumped forward over the steering wheel. When Reg returned he and Leo were able to move him across into the passenger seat but it was clear that he was seriously ill. His left arm was limp and his face contorted. Nothing daunted, he insisted that he should be taken on his Christmas round, delivering presents to friends and associates as though all was well.

What was going through the mind of that tough old brute at that time I can only guess. His greatest fear had

41

always been that he would have to spend his last years in a wheelchair. 'I'd like to die at the wheel of a racing car,' he used to say, and then add, 'at the age of seventy.'

Daddy remembered being called from his office after they got back home. The housekeeper's voice was agitated. 'Please come at once. Your father has had a stroke,' she said. Donald rushed to Little Gatton. The curtains in Malcolm's room were partly drawn, and in the half-light Father tip-toed across the room. As he did so the old man turned towards him; it was a stark, tragic, heartrending sight. This vital, dynamic, colourful figure lay with the left side of his face paralysed and his left arm drooping like a dead branch.

All that remained of the former fire was the recognition in his eyes. Daddy recalled, 'As though pole-axed, I fell on my knees.' He must have been in tears, for he remembers that with his still healthy right hand, Malcolm took Dad's handkerchief from his jacket and wiped his eyes – as perhaps he had done many years before. As he did so he haltingly whispered, 'I'm done for, old boy – finished.'

Grandfather hung on grimly. He had been looking forward so much to a family get-together on Christmas Day. My father and mother and Jean, my aunt, tried to conceal the date, but the nurse let the cat out of the bag and there was a brief glimpse of the old man's determination. 'I do hate being taken for a bloody fool,' he stumbled out in just audible terms, 'fetch a bottle of champagne.' Doing their best to put a brave face on this strange Christmas toast, the family held high their glasses of champagne, and in faltering hand Grandfather raised his glass of medicine. Soon afterwards he relapsed into a coma, and died just before midnight on New Year's Eve. He was laid to rest with my great-grandparents in St Nicholas Churchyard, in Chislehurst.

Leaving the funeral, my father's mind went back to a warm September afternoon in 1897 of which he had been told. A boy with his hands in his pockets careered down Chislehurst Hill, not far from that churchyard, on a bicycle. He hurtled under the railway bridge, scaring the life out of two elderly ladies who were about to cross the road. When he stopped, the local constable was soon on the scene and the offender was charged with furious riding. In court was a crusty old magistrate who glared sternly over his spectacles and said, 'Fined ten shillings, and let this be a lesson to you not to go so fast in future, Malcolm Campbell.'

Between that court appearance and the funeral Malcolm Campbell inscribed his name in the history of sport and engineering as few other men had done. He was one of the first men to be captivated by the possibilities of flying. He was a courageous, single-minded character, with a forceful personality. 'You could love him, you could hate him,' they said, 'but you could never forget him.'

Our family is, of course, Scottish, hailing from the clan Campbell of Argyll. One of my ancestors – in company with 3,000 of his kinsmen – bore arms for Bonnie Prince Charlie. In 1745 the Scottish clans massed and, after an initial victory at Flodden Field, they were routed at the bloody battle of Culloden. Massacre and persecution followed the English victory.

Lord Campbell escaped with his life, but dispossessed of his lands, he wandered the Highlands with a price on his head. In 1757 King James II restored the right to wear the tartan which had been prohibited, on pain of death, since the battle of Flodden Field. My forebear, Lord Campbell, settled down in Tain and died there in 1776.

One relic of those tempestuous days – a strange one to find in the home of a girl – has been handed down to me. It's a broadsword. I value it highly. Being the end of the line, I have to be both son and daughter in a family dominated by strong males. The blade was fashioned by the famous Italian swordmaker Andrea Ferrara. The

43

steel is so finely tempered that it is still possible to bend the point round the hilt. It is an impressive weapon and I still feel family pride in showing it off to friends who visit me.

It was my great-great-great-grandfather who decided to leave Scotland. In fact, he walked the 600 miles from Tain to London. As though to prove the fighting spirit of the Campbells, no sooner had he arrived than he joined the Duke of Wellington's army and fought at the battle of Waterloo. He was mentioned in dispatches and awarded a very imposing-looking medal which sadly disappeared soon after Malcolm Campbell died and has never been traced.

After the Iron Duke's victory, this Campbell founded a firm of diamond merchants in the City of London. The business prospered through three generations and finally passed out of our family on the death of my great-grandfather in 1920. It is strange to think that the financial base which enabled Grandfather, as a private individual, to attain worldwide speed prowess in cars and boats was laid so long before the internal combustion engine was invented.

My great-grandfather, William Campbell, who was the last member of our family in the diamond business, was an astute, industrious man with a broad sense of humour and kind disposition, to judge from all accounts. He was intensely fond of travel. At the age of forty-two he married seventeen-year-old Ada. The difference in their ages lends some substance to the story that at one time he had been courting her widowed mother. Though beautiful, Ada turned out to be insular, narrow-minded and selfish.

William and Ada had two children – the sweet, kind and gentle Freda, and my grandfather, Malcolm. The family lived surrounded by Victoriana in a splendid house on the edge of Chislehurst Common. Both children loved horses and became fine riders, and I am happy to have inherited that love.

44

Malcolm Campbell went to a prep school near Guildford, in Surrey. The gruesome stories he delighted to tell even in adult life about the floggings, burnings and beatings which went on made the place sound as though it could have been the setting for *Oliver Twist*, my father said.

From Guildford, Malcolm went to Uppingham School, situated in what was then Rutland, the smallest county in England. It was a rough, tough, traditional public school. Two weeks after arriving, 'new nips', as the new boys were called, had to sit an examination set by the House Proposters, or 'pollies', as they were known. It was quite an ordeal. Candidates were asked to name past housemasters and captains, state the order of precedence of the rugby and cricket teams' colours, and name the reigning captains of rugby, cricket, shooting, fives and boxing. To pass was all but impossible as there was no established source of information, and the older boys were certainly not telling. Strokes of the cane or a beating with a plimsoll were the price of failure.

Later Daddy also went to Uppingham, but by his time the system had been somewhat tempered, though he still thought it was odd that boys' parents paid vast sums in school fees to have their sons treated like slaves for the first couple of years they were at school. On reflection he came to feel that the rigour of public school life taught a boy to be independent and conscious of the needs of others. With a twinkle in his eye he would also add, 'It ensures that, at some time in his career, every bully is himself bullied.'

Two interests which were to shape his whole life became evident while my grandfather was at Uppingham. One was his interest in things mechanical, the other his lust for adventure. Together they almost led to disaster. One morning after prayers the headmaster announced that a boy had been given twenty-four strokes of the cane after being caught walking through the nearby Glaston railway tunnel. In forceful terms he made it clear

45

that anyone repeating such a foolhardy act would be punished in the same way and expelled.

Such a prohibition was a challenge to Malcolm. Next afternoon, dressed in running kit, he and a companion found their way to Glaston tunnel, hitching a lift on a shunting engine on the way. With their daredevil instinct at its highest peak they walked through a cutting to the tunnel entrance. Once inside, they were soon in darkness, stumbling in their light running shoes over the sleepers and the ballast. Undeterred, they made good progress and felt that they had all but reached the midway point when they heard the sound of a distant train. In their planning they had omitted to check the timetable to see when trains passed through the tunnel. The distant sound became a rumbling and the tracks began to vibrate. Behind them the line was clear, ahead there was a bend so they could not see on which track the train was travelling. They were trapped: there was nothing for it but to stand in the middle and wait. In the eerie darkness the rumble became a roar. The temptation to run was almost irresistible but they stood their ground.

Suddenly, with a shattering crescendo of sound, the lights of the engine came into sight. With the thundering train no more than yards from them they leapt across the track which it was not using and pressed themselves in terror against the wall of the tunnel. The ground shook, the walls shuddered, they were choked with smoke and steam, and covered in soot. The paralysing terror passed and a brash bravado took over, though circumstances denied them the satisfaction of talking of their experience at supper back at school.

Like so many other great men, Malcolm Campbell's scholastic attainments failed to match up to the high standards of the school to which he was sent. An undistinguished school record didn't hinder Sir Winston Churchill and neither did it my grandfather. I sometimes wonder whether our schools are not geared to producing average people, rather than bringing out individual qualities. The result is that the mediocre and conventional are applauded, while the exceptional is only tolerated. In my own upbringing, and that of my father, there was what I think of as the ideal balance between discipline and freedom; the encouragement to take risks and accept challenges on the clear understanding that we had to accept the consequences ourselves if things went wrong, neither making excuses nor blaming someone else. It is a hard philosophy, but it is a better preparation for living than the narrow academic curriculum of many schools.

This does not mean that I think the study of basic subjects and passing examinations is to be despised, but rather to say that, on the evidence of my own family in recent generations, more has been learned outside the classroom than within it. I do not have any children and have no particular desire to be a mother, but I wish parents, teachers and those who organise education would recognise the values of teaching aimed at making people complete as human beings rather than cogs to fit into a slot. I lost count of the number of schools to which I went and the number of times that Dad turned up at school and said, 'Come on, we're flying over to France,' or, 'Get yourself ready, you're off to America with me tomorrow.' The result is that I have few paper qualifications, apart from my secretarial certificate. But I have more than most people to offer, I believe, as a result of my travels and the emotional earthquakes with which I have had to cope, mostly alone.

When Malcolm Campbell left Uppingham he spent four months touring with his father in the Middle East. William Campbell thought it was important for his son to see something of the world. Afterwards, he went to Germany, spending a year in a small hotel on the outskirts of Neubrandenburg learning the language and studying engineering.

Neubrandenburg is a lakeside town surrounded by

forest, and it provided an ideal setting in which the young Malcolm could prove his independence. The rigid structures of Uppingham were far away and for the first time he was free from parental control. Yet the Boer War was at its height and to be an Englishman in Germany was a lonely role, for the country was dominated by anti-British feeling at the time.

Fortunately, Grandfather became firm and inseparable friends with Freido Geertz, a young German who lived close to the hotel. Together they shared many adventures. Towards the end of that summer, a hut in the forest which they had been using as a den was inexplicably burnt down. With winter approaching, the two decided that a cave would be a snug alternative. There were no natural caves in the locality so Malcolm and Freido had to excavate one for themselves. They worked very hard digging into the near vertical face of the hillside and before long hollowed out a good sized room. Eager to get the job completed my grandfather decided to continue with the digging on his own one evening. He continued until two in the morning, and then, utterly exhausted, he trudged back to his hotel, more than ready for bed.

I have no idea why he was carrying a revolver, but as he took it off, in his tiredness his finger accidentally touched the trigger. The silence of the night was shattered by the noise of the gun going off, and within minutes the manager of the hotel was hammering on his door demanding in guttural tones an explanation for this outrage. The bullet had grazed Malcolm's temple and gone through the ceiling. He was shattered by the knowledge that had it been pointing a fraction further to the left everyone would have thought that he had committed suicide.

Early next morning Freido turned up looking pale and agitated. After Grandfather had left the cave he had gone there and found that part of the hillside had collapsed. He had spent the rest of the night feverishly

48

clawing at the rocks and soil with his bare hands in an attempt to rescue his friend whom he feared had been trapped. Ironically the next day a letter arrived from my great grandmother imploring Malcolm to give up work on the cave as it was dangerous!

At this stage in his youth my grandfather had a taste for good cigars but he noticed that quite regularly some were being taken from the box in his room. In a spare moment he took a handful, carefully undid the wrapping, removed some of the tobacco in the centre, replaced it with a tiny quantity of explosive, rewound the outer leaves and put them back into the box.

One evening, a few days later, Malcolm wanted to go into Neubrandenburg and booked the hotel horse and buggy to take him, knowing that it would be driven by Hans, the member of the staff whom he thought had been taking his cigars. As he left his room he put the box under his arm and before climbing aboard outside the hotel, with apparent gentlemanly generosity offered Hans a cigar, saying that he would have one later in the town with a drink. Hans gladly accepted, lit up, and they trotted off into the darkness. They had just entered the town square when there was a flash and a bang. Hans remained sitting upright in the driving seat, looking straight ahead, his face immobile, with the remains of the shattered cigar clenched between his teeth. He was the picture of Germanic equanimity. Grandfather said not a word but no more of his cigars disappeared.

All too soon, from his point of view, the time came for Malcolm to say *auf wiedersehen*, but not before he had bought his first bicycle. It was a not particularly good second-hand one, but with it he showed his competitive nature for the first time. He entered himself in a closed circuit professional cycling race. Although lacking experience as a cyclist, and knowing nothing of professional cycling, he finished third. By anyone's standards it was a creditable performance, but for Grandfather winning was the only ground for satisfaction in any competition.

Back in Chislehurst he found the routines of home life restrictive. Discipline teaches people how to use freedom, but if ever personal freedom is then replaced by an imposed discipline it is irksome. Matters came to a head one evening after supper. Malcolm was writing a letter to his girlfriend of the moment, an attractive and much sought after young lady who was the daughter of the local squire. For some reason his mother did not approve of the friendship and, knowing what he was doing, persuaded her husband to order Malcolm to bed. William Campbell gave the required instructions. 'Very well, sir,' said Malcolm, 'I'll just finish this letter.' With that his father lost his temper. 'How dare you bandy words with me? To bed, this instant,' he shouted. With that the old man strode to the centre of the room and took hold of the chain to extinguish the gaslight. Grandfather jumped up and seized the chain on the opposite side of the mantle, and a see-saw developed. The light spluttered and went dim, then burned brightly, went dim again, and then shone brightly once more. Even a Victorian gas fitting was not designed to withstand such treatment; the fitting pulled away from the ceiling, the centre rose and its surrounding plaster decorating William Campbell's head. The following morning the errant son packed his bags and left and, although soon reconciled to his father, he was never to live at home again.

4

During the last few months of Malcolm's stay in Germany, his father had written again and again, asking him to make up his mind about a job. The exhortations had little effect, and neither did a short spell in France do anything to clarify his thinking. He seems to have been content to seek out personal challenges for himself and indulge in the pleasures of life which were available to an energetic young man from a well-to-do background without much thought of anyone else.

This was intolerable to his parents, and while he was briefly living at home, after his return from the continent, his father apprenticed him to Messrs Tizer & Co., who were insurance brokers at Lloyd's. Travelling by train from Chislehurst into London and back each day was far removed from the life he had enjoyed in Germany or the adventures which were to dominate his future years. He did well, and recorded that he earned fifteen shillings a week. Within four years, in 1906, as a twenty-first birthday present, William Campbell entered his son in partnership in the firm of Pitman & Dean. This made him a Lloyd's underwriter.

For a time business was bleak, but suddenly my grandfather's genius showed through. A London newspaper covered a sporting event in France through the eyes of an imaginary holidaymaker who spent much of his time drinking and womanising. Unfortunately for the paper the pseudonym it gave its fictional reporter was the name of a real person. The man took legal action and was awarded £1,750 damages. Malcolm immediately saw the need for newspapers to insure themselves against libel.

It was a totally new concept and not one readily accepted either by Lloyds underwriters or the newspapers. Eventually he formulated an insurance policy which was approved by Lloyd's, and then spent day after day climbing creaky stairs and visiting the musty offices of Fleet Street. The first company to commit itself to the new cover was known then as Odham, Southwood & Co., but gradually others followed suit.

It was characteristic of my grandfather that he never allowed business problems or successes to deflect him for long from his sporting interests. While he was working on his new insurance venture he bought a three-and-a-half horsepower Quadrant motorcycle. He entered the London to Land's End Trial – which was an important national event in those days – and won it. It was his first among many trophies, but his friends said it was just a fluke. To prove them wrong he took part in the trial again in 1907 and 1908, and won again on both occasions.

He had been invited to see a film about the Wright brothers' experiments with heavier-than-air flying machines during 1903. Wilbur and Orville Wright's aeroplane was seen as the most exciting invention ever. Grandfather was captivated. Seeing that film was one of the landmarks of his life. Outside business hours he thought of little else but flying, and in his lunchtimes would stand day after day on London Bridge, seeing again Wrights' first flight, his eyes watching the seagulls effortlessly soaring and wheeling. The freedom of the limitless sky fascinated him, and he was convinced that this was the sphere man would conquer.

While Malcolm was dreaming Louis Blériot and Hubert Latham were waiting for favourable weather so that they could make the first attempt to fly across the English Channel. Latham tried first but his plane crashed into the sea, and many people felt that the Channel could never be crossed by air. Grandfather felt differently. He had been reading everything available on the theory of flight, studying drawings and photographs of existing machines, and building models. So confident was he that Blériot would succeed, that he arranged an insurance policy at Lloyd's against the risk of Blériot's success.

On 25 July 1909 Blériot flew the Channel and landed at Dover. Most people were impressed by the clichéd headline 'Dawn of new era'; Grandfather collected £750 from the insurance he had taken out and used it to continue his own experiments in flying.

By this time, the desire to fly was an obsession with Malcolm. When Blériot's plane was on display in an Oxford Street store, in London, he went to see it again and again, each time sketching parts and making notes on how it had been built. He heard about a display of aircraft and flying to take place at Reims, in France. Such was his enthusiasm that when the ferry on which he was crossing from England ran aground near the French coast, threatening to make him miss the opening, he begged a lift on a small boat which came out from the harbour and reached Reims just in time to see the President of France open the show. Somehow, he and the friend who had travelled with him managed to infiltrate the official party on its tour of the display stands and so were able to get an excellent view of everything.

Spurred on by a cash prize of £1,000 offered by a newspaper to the first Englishman to fly, Grandfather decided to build a plane. He rented a barn on the edge of a strawberry field in Kent and engaged a full-time carpenter. Each evening, when he returned from the City, he would go straight to the field and begin work. Often they were there until three in the morning, and night after night their meal consisted of beer and sandwiches. The only visitor they ever had was the local policeman. He appreciated the warmth of the brazier on winter nights and enjoyed a sandwich and a beer. Malcolm encouraged his visits as it was becoming increasingly clear that a number of local people were hostile to the venture. We laugh at the thought of people saying it nowadays, but plenty then seriously believed that if God had intended man to fly He would have given him wings – so the new-fangled flying machines could only be the invention of the devil, and the local people wanted none of it near their community.

Sooner than Grandfather expected the money he had made at Lloyd's on Blériot's flight was gone, and he had to raise more by selling his car. Slowly his aeroplane took shape. It was a copy of Blériot's with a twin cylinder two-and-a-half horsepower Jap engine taken from a motor bike. Two bicycle wheels served as undercarriage, and one from a pram was the tail skid.

He selected a Sunday in June for the trial flight, but when Malcolm, his carpenter, and two friends who had come along to help push out the new machine from the barn they were met by a large and hostile crowd. The village constable was nowhere to be seen!

The objectors decided that the most effective way to prevent the aircraft taking off was to form an unbroken line across the field. Grandfather pleaded with them to move, but they refused. It was neck or nothing, he felt. He was not going to have his great moment marred by a mob of villagers who had neither the wit to appreciate his vision nor the tolerance to allow someone else to do what they would never have the guts to attempt themselves.

Malcolm climbed into the cockpit, the two friends held the wings and the carpenter swung the propeller. Up to that moment Malcolm had believed that the noise of the engine would scare his adversaries into retreat. There was a gradual movement backwards but they were still determined. The scene must have been comic. Grandfather was perched on top of the fragile contraption, which resembled a cross between a prehistoric kite and a Victorian bedstead, while the villagers shouted their objections.

When the engine had warmed up my grandfather decided that there was just enough distance between him and the crowd for the plane to reach its take-off speed and become airborne. He opened the throttle, the men at the wing tips let go, and the machine rumbled and bounced down the field.

The plane was accelerating, but at a much lower rate than expected. It began to loom dangerously close to the crowd but they still showed no sign of moving. The situation was desperate; the machine had no brakes, the objectors were standing their ground, and Grandfather had no alternative but to pull back the joystick in the hope of avoiding killing or injuring many of the people. 'By the mercy of God,' as he put it, 'the plane shuddered into the air, just clear of the heads of the misguided crowd.'

Almost at once it stalled and flopped to the ground. All those long nights of hard work had produced a heap of junk just a couple of hundred yards from the place where the contraption had been put together. My grandfather emerged from the mass of splintered wood and broken wires to the jeers of the villagers and the problem of getting the wreckage back to the barn. There he and his friends found their jackets had been rifled and everything stolen.

Repair work on the damaged plane had less appeal than the original construction. Grandfather bought new parts, up-to-date propellers and a more powerful engine but the fragile craft never stayed in the air for more than a few seconds and certainly never managed to clear the hedge at the end of the field. By this time he was dispirited and without money so he decided to try to sell the plane and start from scratch again.

Frizwells, who were well-known London car dealers, persuaded Malcolm to allow them to sell his aircraft. It would be the first time an aeroplane had been offered at auction, they said. The idea appealed to my grandfather. Bidding was brisk, but at £270 there was a pause. Malcolm decided to try to help things along and said. 'And ten.' The pause became an ominous silence with the auctioneer desperately trying to raise another bid. 'Going . . . going . . . gone.' He had bought his own plane. At once he approached the last bidder, only to be told, 'You bought it, you bloody keep it.' The net result was a bill for the commission of £25 10s. And that was exactly the price the plane made when it went under the hammer again a day or two later.

Broke, and with insufficient knowledge to make a go of flying, Malcolm Campbell decided to turn his attention to motor racing. Brooklands, which was the mecca of British motor racing from the time it was built in 1904 until 1939, was near Weybridge, not too far from his home in Reigate. The two-and-three-quarter-mile track consisted of two long straights connected by very highly banked curves. The place is a sad sight now. Much of it has become an industrial estate. When I went there in 1987, to see where Grandfather had raced, the security man was only interested in keeping me away from soulless factory units and couldn't appreciate that for me the place is part of my family heritage. Perhaps it was just as well, though. The track where my grandfather first gave vent to his passion for mechanical excellence and thrilled a generation with his pursuit of speed now has elder and blackberries growing though cracks in the concrete, among abandoned old cookers and discarded mattresses.

Driving racing cars at Brooklands, and the fact that his business life at Lloyds was beginning to develop well, helped to mollify Malcolm's anger at not managing to build a plane and fly it himself. His anger was not that of a disappointed child who has been denied but the frustration of a strong man who has not been able to achieve his ambition because of factors outside his control. In his case he had neither the money nor the know-how to construct a flying machine that would live up to its name. Time passed and he spent hours brooding until he realised that he had to accept that he was not destined to be a pioneer of aviation.

Already he had driven at Brooklands in a rather light-hearted way. On a gala day in 1908 he had finished a long way behind the leading pack, and later that year he had the use of a twin cylinder Renault which had completed the Paris/Madrid race in 1903 but had finished nowhere. It was a 4.9 litre Darracq – a formidable machine weighing more than a ton and capable of over 80 mph – which gave him his first real success in motor racing. In next to no time his morose mood of failure was transformed into a determination to win a classic planned for Brooklands on August Bank Holiday.

Grandfather's ruthless approach to any competition was quickly evident. He decided that a Peugeot would give him a better chance of being first across the line than the massive Darracq. Despite his shortage of money he acquired one and, following the fashion of that time, gave it a nickname – it was to be The Flapper. He might well have chosen more wisely. The original Flapper was a horse with an unusually long tail which was running at Kempton Park. A colleague at Lloyds, who owned and backed horses, persuaded him to put some money on it. He had already learned that gambling was not something at which he – or many other people, for that matter – made a profit, but the name appealed to him. It used to amuse him to pull the pigtails of his flapper cousins. Some money went on the horse and its name went on the Peugeot, but to say that the horse was an also ran would have been to overestimate its achievement. The car finished well down the field too.

Someone told Grandfather of another Darracq which was said to be capable of 100 mph. When he went to see it, it was in the middle of a junk yard in Kennington and he had to clear masses of debris away before he could really make an assessment of the vehicle. It turned out to be a really formidable machine with cylinders over six inches in diameter. It had a full tank and the tyres were pumped up so it was ready for the road, but it was some minutes before either of his colleagues was prepared to turn the beast's crank handle. On a somewhat impatient word from my grandfather one of the men did the necessary and the engine roared into life. Malcolm eased the magnificent car out of the yard and it was on its way to his home of that time at Sundridge Park, near Bromley. A drive along the roads of suburban London in those days before the First World War was a dusty business but my grandfather was perched high with pride, convinced that he had a winner this time.

The old machine was overhauled and spruced up, and given the name Flapper II. She won her first race at Brooklands and was entered for the classic. On the evening before the big race Malcolm went out to dinner in London and then on to the theatre to see Maeterlinck's play *The Bluebird*. It is the fable of the elusive Bluebird of happiness which is by the side of each of us, always within reach and yet, if pursued, always beyond our grasp.

Grandfather was enthralled by the play – and most of all by the title. 'Here, surely,' he thought, 'was the only name suitable for the new Darracq.' His companion was as understanding as she was lovely, and willingly agreed to forego the customary after-theatre supper. The lady was safely delivered to her home with minimal courtesies and Grandfather dashed home to Sundridge Park. On the way he dragged the local ironmonger out of bed, buying every tin of blue paint he had in his shop along with a quantity of turpentine and some brushes. The painting of the car took until four o'clock in the morning. The new colour scheme was finally complete and he drove the car, with the paintwork still tacky, to Brooklands in time for the race. That day the first Bluebird appeared before the public. There was a large colourful crowd and an atmosphere charged with excitement, for many of the closer followers of motor racing knew well of Grandfather's dedication to winning this Brooklands classic.

The formalities complete, the flag fell for the start of the big race. The Darracq went into the lead at once, then lost it, then struggled back into the lead again, and finally and gloriously went through to win. Bluebird was first across the line! Grandfather was ecstatic. The name which has become synonymous with speed on both land and water, with daring and courage, with care and hazard, with record breaking and eventually with tragedy, was for the first time lightly etched on a page of British sporting history that August day.

In preparing to write this book I came across some pages which my father, Donald Campbell, had intended as the basis of his own book but which never got beyond the stage of being a draft. He reflected on the name Bluebird and in more than twenty years no one read what he wrote. It sums up not only what the name of successive cars and boats has meant but the way of thinking which unites and has inspired my grandfather, my father and now me. I am proud to quote what Dad wrote as the Preface to my book.

Later in the same year Bluebird was entered for another race at Brooklands. Just before she was pushed to the line a well-wisher gave my grandfather a small black toy cat as a mascot. Whether its presence proved to be a good omen or not is open to doubt.

Because of her previous victory, Bluebird was heavily handicapped, but came off the banking on the last lap lying in fourth place though doing 100 mph. She was set fair to catch the leader but at that moment the offside front tyre burst. The car lurched into a violent skid and was almost sideways across the track. It took all my grandfather's giant strength to correct her course and, determined to win, he kept his foot hard down on the accelerator. She was almost back on line when the damaged wooden wheel struck a low concrete curb and shattered into a thousand fragments. The largest part of it skimmed over the head of a track attendant while the rim bent and twisted the iron railing he was standing behind. Bluebird was completely out of control.

The crowd were massed on the other side of the railings and only Grandfather seemed to be aware of the danger they were in. With all the muscle power at his disposal he pulled the steering wheel to full opposite lock, knowing that the strain could break the linkage and the car could plunge headlong into the people with unthinkable consequences. Yet none of the spectators made any attempt to run. It was as though they were mesmerised by the awesome sight of one man doing battle with a motorised raging bull. I have seen this kind of thing happen again and again. Onlookers at a sporting event in which there are high risks involved do not want to see participants killed, but it is part of the adrenalin-stimulating entertainment that there are moments when it seems as if disaster will occur. Strangest of all is that at such moments the people who are watching may be in equal or even greater danger, yet their thoughts and emotions are so much projected onto the event that few will sense the danger and panic.

At Brooklands the linkage did break but miraculously Bluebird lurched further out onto the track before again turning towards the crowd. By this time she had lost some of her impetus, bounced off another concrete curb and over the finishing line. She was placed fourth!

In that irrational way that even the strongest of men have, Grandfather blamed the mascot which he had been given for the mishap, picked up the little black cat from between the seats of the car and threw it into a ditch. Hours later, as the full impact of the narrowness of his escape and the realisation of what a disaster could have taken place began to dawn on him, he went back to the spot where the car had come to a standstill and recovered the black cat. My father remembers the cat had a prominent place in Grandfather's garage for the rest of his life. Sadly, it was stolen – presumably by a souvenir hunter – soon after Grandfather died.

Bluebird was repaired, but she never again showed her former speed. She was the first of a line which was to conquer the world as far as records were concerned.

Motor racing had to take second place in my grandfather's life during the next few years: like thousands of others he rushed to join up as soon as war was declared in 1914. He applied for a commission in the Royal West Kent Regiment but, impatient with administrative delays and convinced that the war would be over before he reached the front, he enlisted as a motorcycle dispatch rider. In those days, I'm told, motorcyclists were few and far between and his services were readily accepted.

He was at the battle of Mons where the conflict was particularly intense and positions changed hands rapidly. One evening he was dispatched with a message to battalion headquarters in a café on the edge of a small village. He had already been there several times that day. In the gathering dusk he was about to draw up and dismount when he was horrified to be greeted by men in coal-scuttle helmets. It was a lively if inhospitable welcome. Fortunately he was quickly off down the road, his backside concealed by a cloud of dust and small stones, but followed by a hail of bullets.

When his commission in the Royal West Kents came through he served with them for about a year but was then seconded to the Royal Flying Corps. This unexpected turn of fortune made it possible for him to fulfil his ambition of years before and learn to fly, this time at someone else's expense. Flying training was sketchy by modern standards, and after only two hours of instruction at Gosport he made his first solo flight. He was awarded his wings when he had had just ten hours' flying experience. My grandfather's first posting as a pilot was to a ferry unit. His job was to fly new aeroplanes to France and return with damaged ones which were somewhat pessimistically marked 'unfit for further flying'.

Donald told me once that he had not appreciated how hairy one of Grandfather's experiences was until he himself learned to fly some forty years later. Apparently one day Grandfather had flown two new machines from Lydd, in Kent, to St Omer, in France, and brought two others back for repair. As he crossed the Channel with a third new aircraft there was a heavy bank of mist developing along the French coast near Dunkirk. He landed safely at St Omer late in the evening and was once again asked to take a damaged plane back to England. It had been more seriously knocked about than the earlier ones but after the appropriate checks he was allowed to fly it. He began his homeward journey but the mist-covered area had extended, and the first time he knew anything about crossing the French coast was when he cleared the mist and found himself to be already over the sea.

Instruments on aircraft in those early days of flying were of a most rudimentary nature; there was no radio contact, and no navigational aids. With little more than a simple map and guesswork to guide him he decided to make for Calais aerodrome and hope for the best. At 1,000 feet he and his machine entered a thick, grey wall of fog. As he kept going his altimeter went down and down; at 500 feet he gave up hope and sat there waiting for the end. The needle continued to drop – 400, 300, 200 and then zero. At that moment, out of the gloom, two large lumps appeared straight ahead of him. He knew them. They were the hangars at the edge of Calais aerodrome. They were too close together for him to glide between them so he banked steeply in an attempt to skirt around them, but he had lost his flying speed. It was too late and his aircraft crashed. Malcolm was badly shaken by this crash, though not seriously hurt. My father used to reckon that it was one of the narrowest escapes of his hazard-filled life.

After some leave he served as an instructor in the Royal Flying Corps and then spent some time hunting Zeppelins. It says a great deal for the fitness of my grandfather and his colleagues that they sustained such a patrol at a height of between 16,000 and 17,000 feet without oxygen.

Just before the war ended Grandfather was flying a Bristol freighter and his oldest and dearest friend, Donald Hay, was piloting a similar machine in parallel. They began to practise some aerobatics and dog fights when, without warning, the wings of Donald Hay's machine folded up and it plummeted to the earth like a falling stone. Hay was killed instantly. Grandfather vowed that if ever he had a son he would be christened Donald.

Service life with its discipline, challenges and clearly understood structures of rank and responsibility suited Grandfather, and he delighted – as he had every right to do – in continuing to use the rank of captain before his name in civilian life when the war ended. He returned to Lloyds and also set himself up quite successfully in the motor trade, holding the British agencies for several of the more exclusive continental cars of the time. He drove in every race for which he was eligible at Brooklands, and there and elsewhere he won a mass of trophies. As a racing driver he was beginning to stand out from the rest but, tiring of Brooklands, he determined in 1922 that he would tackle the Land Speed Record.

Leo Villa joined Grandfather as his racing mechanic at this stage, and began an association which was to be essential to both Malcolm and Donald. Leo had been working for the Italian racing driver and businessman, Giulio Foresti, in Paris and came with him to deliver a car which Malcolm had bought. Leo had received a letter from Grandfather before he left Paris suggesting that he might join him as his mechanic and offering him a wage of £3 a week. On the way from Folkestone to Surrey, where by this time Grandfather lived, Malcolm took over the controls of the Ballot car which Leo had been driving. It seems that as well as sizing up the car he was sizing up Leo. Did he smoke or drink? Grandfather asked. Did he go with women? How interested was he in motor racing? Leo was shrewd enough to know a spontaneous job interview when he was in one, and to recognise that his would-be employer did not have the easy charm which he so much appreciated in Foresti. But Leo had lived out of a suitcase for long enough, and longed to be back in England and closer to other members of his family, so he took the job. But the escape from the suitcase life was not as complete as he had anticipated.

Grandfather's workshop and garage were at Povey Cross, a five-hundred-year-old country house which, so they said, had once been the home of the highwayman Dick Turpin. The cowshed had been converted into the base from which Malcolm's racing operation was run. Leo's first impression was of spotless and meticulous tidiness. The workshop was light and airy, with an enormous bench along one wall. On that bench, laid out with military precision, were all the tools a man could ever need. The walls were covered with photographs of famous racing cars and Leo felt that here he could be happy and do an efficient job.

Before Leo Villa accepted the post Malcolm laid down his rules. 'I'm a stickler for tidiness,' he said, 'and if you join me, I insist that the workshop is kept in the state it is now.' Grandfather's military bearing came out in so much he did. He liked a job to be done in double quick time and was never really happy if the tools were out of their proper place for too long. And if anyone got oil or grease on the floor, which is inevitable in a workshop, it had to be wiped up smartly or there was trouble.

Unlike Foresti, who was always under the cars himself and taught Leo most of what he knew about being a mechanic, my Grandfather preferred to go shooting, work in the fields around the house, or care for the Airedales he was breeding at the time, or his horse. This was one of the big differences between Grandfather and Father. Dad was a mechanic and engineer in his own right and was involved as much in the planning, building and maintenance sides of his record breaking as he was in the driving. Grandfather could talk cars with anyone, but when it came to the practical side he was not very handy. Leo said in his book *The Record Breakers*, 'If there was a job to be done that required two pairs of hands, I preferred to ask anyone rather than the Skipper.' Foresti's reaction to almost anything had been calm and light-hearted, but quickly Leo Villa recognised that Malcolm Campbell was going to be a difficult boss. He wrote, 'With Campbell there was always a feeling of tension. I was going to do my best for him, I always did anyway, but the feeling of tension was an added responsibility . . . I wasn't ever told precisely what my duties were to be, either. I was officially purely a racing mechanic, but if Campbell said to me: "Villa, will you have a look at the Rolls, old boy," you can bet your life that old boy would have a look.'

5

Becoming a champion, or a record breaker, requires unusually advanced skills, whatever the area of human achievement involved. Equally, it demands an attitude of mind and qualities of temperament which set the champion-to-be apart from every rival. To what extent I have these attributes is not for me to say. Certainly if you had seen me on the day I achieved my own world record you'd have said I have them to the full, but within myself I know there is an element of bluff about my super-confident approach to both record breaking and powerboat racing. Inside me there are questionings and uncertainties, and I suspect that both Grandfather and Father knew a similar soul-searching, before a major challenge. It is equally true that they had – and I share their determination – a passion to be the best at everything they did, and to win any competition in which they entered. In ordinary day-to-day driving I am content to potter along comfortably as long as there is an empty road ahead of me, but if another car appears, I cannot resist taking it on until I am ahead of it. Similarly, like Malcolm, in my home I have the pedantic need to be tidy.

Even in his early racing days at Brooklands, Grandfather was sometimes guilty of stealing a second or two by getting across the starting line before the flag went down. Ebby Ebblewhite, the official timekeeper at Brooklands in those days, was used to Malcolm's starts and would simply make an addition to his handicap. Grandfather gained a reputation at Brooklands, and if he didn't win, the newspaper headlines the next day would read 'Campbell beaten into Second Place'. That he could not tolerate. There was betting on the course, too, and he faced additional pressure because he was invariably the favourite and hated to let himself down.

Two other factors marked out Captain Malcolm Campbell, as he was then, from other drivers. One was his independence; other aspirants to the World Land Speed Record gladly accepted cars designed, built and financed by motor companies, but Malcolm's had to be his own efforts. The second was the speed of his reactions; he had lightning responses to whatever happened whilst he was driving, which gave him a great advantage over other competitors and, on more than one occasion, saved him from injury or death. In an almost prophetic way, he once asked Leo Villa never to allow Donald to take up record breaking, as he believed Dad did not have sharp enough responses to cope with emergencies.

In the days soon after the First World War, life at Povey Cross was near idyllic. Leo Villa recalled how Grandfather would come home from London each evening after business, park his car in the garage, have a chat about what had been going on in the workshop that day, and then hurry across to the house for dinner. Later, Leo would sometimes see Grandfather and Grandmother strolling arm in arm in the garden. To him, it seemed exactly what married life should be. This was, of course, Malcolm's second marriage. Its happiness seemed to be complete when their son, who was to be my father, was born on 21 March 1921. In keeping with the vow he made earlier, the baby was christened Donald after Grandfather's great friend Donald Hay.

As the bug to be the fastest man on earth took its hold, more and more pressure was put on the family relationships. Not only was Malcolm away a great deal, but his obsession with speed took on such proportions that his home life was, in the end, completely neglected. Grandfather's first attempt on the World Land Speed Record was in 1922. He believed that a 350 hp Sunbeam, in which Kenelm Lee Guinness had reached 129 mph at Brooklands, could do better on a less cramped track. On the beach at Saltburn, in Yorkshire, he took it up to 135 mph, but the record did not count as the official timekeepers were not there. Never mind, his passion to be the record holder was in the open and never again would he be free of his slavery to speed. Within months, Grandfather bought the Sunbeam and she became the next in the Bluebird line.

The outcome of the International Speed Trials at Fanö, in Denmark, the following year, was again bitter-sweet. No other car could match Bluebird but the timing system was not of a design approved by the Commission Sportive, which had to authenticate all records. Grandfather knew that he had done well, but sometimes in driving there are private satisfactions which do not coincide with setting new world records, or winning trophies. Malcolm had his own way of displaying this sense of personal achievement. Normally he would call Leo Villa just by his surname, as gentry did their employees in those days, but when he was particularly happy with the way things had gone, Leo remembered that Grandfather would come up to him, pat him on the cheek and say, 'Good old Leo!' It happened on a number of occasions and right at the end of his life, just before Malcolm lapsed into a coma, Leo went to see his old boss for the last time, and in a frail voice he said again, 'Good old Leo!' I find this gratifying, because both Grandfather and Father owed more to Leo than anyone else, in what they did and what they were. As an engineer he was brilliant beyond compare, as a man he was unassuming to a fault.

At Fanö a single strand of rope separated the spectators from the track, and before he left Malcolm told the organisers that it was inadequate, as people pushed forward at the most exciting moments, putting themselves and the drivers at risk. How much that warning was needed was proved all too tragically on his next visit there. Bluebird lost a tyre at full speed and it bounced into the crowd, killing a boy who was watching. Naturally, the spectators were incensed, and Grandfather was arrested and charged with manslaughter. When he appeared in court, the magistrates acquitted him and thanked him for the warning he had given, and they rebuked the organisers very severely for failing to heed what he had said.

Very often Malcolm would ask the timekeepers to be in position even though he was not planning to attack the record. Well, that's what he said. It was really a form of bluff. If his speed exceeded the existing record, he could then say that it would have been higher if he had been making a serious effort; if it didn't there was no loss of face. I have learned that there has to be an element of cunning in public relations, or everyone will devalue a great moment by anticipating it!

There was this element about my grandfather's first record. The team had been working on Bluebird and waiting for the right weather at Pendine Sands, in South Wales, for several weeks when Malcolm's patience snapped – or so it seemed. Without fuss or warning he took her out onto the beach and went through the measured mile at 146.16 mph. Not long afterwards he was back at Pendine again to coax an extra mile or two an hour out of Bluebird, and at this point he became the first man to travel at more than 150 mph.

Restless as ever, Grandfather immediately set his sights on doing three miles a minute. It was a challenging landmark and he would need another car if he were to pass it. Design plans which he and a number of friends had in mind were soon off the drawing board, and he persuaded the Air Ministry to lend him a Napier Lion 450 hp engine which was more powerful than any he had used before. Construction work began at Povey Cross with confidence and enthusiasm, but competition for the kudos of holding the World Land Speed Record was hotting up.

Henry Seagrave and Parry Thomas were setting the pace, and Seagrave was to become the hated but necessary rival on land and, later, on water. I say hated but that is really too strong a word. It is human nature that when someone outdoes you in a competitive pursuit you react against them, but their achievement quickly becomes a stimulant to you to make greater efforts yourself, and that's the sort of attitude which my grandfather had towards Seagrave. Even so, he was doing so well that it became clear that the new Bluebird, designed to do 180 mph, was going to be out of date before she was finished.

Morale sank to its lowest at Povey Cross, and Grandfather brought in extra helpers to speed up the construction work. Meals for the additional workers were prepared in the house and served in the granary, which put a great deal of pressure on the domestic staff. In fact, the turnover of staff reached almost world record speed! The team worked round the clock to get Bluebird ready, so that night and day there was the clanging of tools as metal was beaten into shape. And by then Grandfather had no thought of, and no conversation about, anything other than the new car and the record which he was going to hold in the face of all-comers. From all accounts, Grandmother was beside herself. She was doing so much, enduring the disruption of her home, yet her place, she felt, was always a supporting one to that of a machine.

Worse was to follow. It sounds laughable, though I am sure it was not at the time with Grandfather present, but when Bluebird was to be taken out for the first time he found there was not enough room for him to get between the seat and steering wheel! So many modifications had been made while the car was being built that the space for the driver had been whittled away.

It was several more months before all the teething troubles were sorted out and Bluebird was able to prove her worth. By then, Henry Seagrave was on his way to the United States and more favourable conditions than Britain could provide, with a car said to be capable of 200 mph. Parry Thomas, who held the record, was watching as Bluebird wrested it from him on 4 February 1927 with a speed of 174.88 mph. At once Thomas decided to make a new bid but tragically was killed in the attempt. Whatever rivalry – or even animosity – there may be between contenders for world records, moments such as these make us aware of how frail we are beside the powerful machines we seek to control and the forces of nature with which we do battle.

The car which Seagrave had taken to Daytona, in Florida, lived up to its designer's expectations and Grandfather could not help but admire Seagrave's achievement, though he was angry that someone else had been first to exceed 180 mph, and now 200 mph. People had attached a strange mystique to the speed of 200 mph. They said that cars would disintegrate or take to the air, or that irreparable damage would be done to the body or mind of the driver. It was rather similar to the way in which later generations have talked about the sound barrier or space travel. It is amazing to me how men and women adorn what they do not understand with a semi-scientific mythology of danger.

An extensive rebuilding of Bluebird was in hand when my grandfather received an invitation from Daytona to attempt to better Henry Seagrave's record there. Early in 1928 the modified car was crated up, and with Grandfather and the team went across the Atlantic on the liner *Berengaria*. The Daytona authorities saw breaking the World Land Speed Record as part of a programme to promote their city as a holiday centre, and two American aspirants to the record – Frank Lockhart and Ray Keech – were there at the same time. At its best Daytona beach is ideal for speed, but after certain wind conditions it is covered in tiny ridges. All three had to wait some days for the surface to be satisfactory, and Malcolm amused his American hosts by regularly cycling along the beach to assess any improvement.

It's no good pretending otherwise, but Grandfather could be a swine when things did not go his way. His Campbell spunk had been aroused enough by Seagrave's achievements, but now that he was pitted against two Americans he was fighting mad to go. His first run was a complete failure, with Bluebird hitting a bump and taking off for a full twenty yards halfway along the ten-mile course. His anger and sense of urgency inspired the team to get the repairs done in double quick time, and out he went a day or two later to test what they had done. In his usual way he asked the timekeepers to be present. With an expression of brutal determination on his rock-like face, he roared away. There had been enough delays and frustrations, he felt. He gave Bluebird full power all the way and did not make the usual stop before the second run. To the amazement of the service crew Bluebird was gone with a deafening roar, and was soon a speck disappearing into the distance. The World Land Speed Record was his again: 206.95 mph. To Grandfather it was as though he had redressed the balance of the War of Independence!

Within weeks Ray Keech pushed the record up again, and what had previously been a deadly rivalry between Seagrave and Grandfather for personal honours became a mission for Britain in which each would prefer the other to hold the record rather than know that it was in the hands of a foreigner.

Malcolm was one of the world's greatest individualists and had only reluctantly accepted the idea of making a record attempt with other drivers competing at Daytona at the same time. Daytona was therefore out, and he had to find an alternative venue for his next effort.

He was recommended to look at a stretch of sand near Timbuctoo, so he bought a light plane and flew to Africa with a former Flying Corps colleague. To go looking for sand in the Sahara sounds like a joke, but Malcolm was at heart an explorer as well as a record breaker. Twice he had gone abroad hunting for hidden treasure. On neither occasion was he successful, but, like a middle-class Micawber, he always believed that something was about to turn up! When they found the suggested location it was at once clear that there was no way to get Bluebird and all the equipment to such a remote place, and, in any case, it was doubtful whether the team could have survived long enough in the arid heat to see the venture through.

On the way home their plane developed engine trouble and they had to ditch just off a West African beach. They managed to pull it above the high tide mark and then realised that they were surrounded by decidedly aggressive local inhabitants. This must have been one of the few occasions on which Grandfather did as he was told. He and his companion were marched several miles to a village settlement and presented to the village chief. Happily he viewed their arrival with cordiality. They were given a meal, which involved dipping their hands into a common cooking pot to get what they could. They were dying of thirst but could not bring themselves to drink from a container which the villagers had also used to wash their feet, hands and faces.

Next morning they were allowed to leave. Over the next two or three days they trekked aimlessly until they came across a Spanish army outpost, where they got helpers to return to the plane with them and make it airworthy for the journey home.

After looking at several other possible sites Grandfather decided on Verneuk Pan, a dried up lake about 450 miles inland from Cape Town, in South Africa. It had seemed an ideal place according to the report of a friend who did the reconnaissance, but when they arrived there early in 1929 they found that the twelve-mile track had to be cleared of sharp splinters of shale and there was little local labour available. There was no accommodation on the site, food had to be brought in from 120 miles away and the nearest water was 12 miles distant. This was my father's first trip to a record attempt, and it should have been a warning to him. He and Jean stayed with their mother and governess in Cape Town, and Grandfather commuted in his Gipsy Moth between there and Verneuk Pan daily. To add to Malcolm's misfortunes, another pilot offered to take them on one trip and, returning to Cape Town, hit a tree and crashed. Grandfather was cut quite badly in a number of places, and suffered serious bruising to his stomach, which kept him out of action for more than a week. During that week, for the first time in years the rains came at Verneuk Pan and the carefully prepared track was destroyed.

My grandfather was a man of military bearing, and never were his qualities of leadership more severely tested than at Verneuk Pan. It was a place that sapped energy and morale, and Malcolm needed to be Captain Campbell in every way possible to keep the team together and maintain the credibility of his challenge. As well as the flags marking the course and the poles indicating the start and the finish of the measured mile, this time he insisted that a 12-inch wide white line should be painted down the full length of the course. This eccentric request was taken by some of the team as a sign that the Skipper's sight was not quite as good as it once had been.

The disappointments and annoyances at Verneuk Pan seemed to be complete when, as the party withdrew, a truck carrying spares crashed into a ravine. For all I know, its rusting wreckage may still be there. For the record book, and in fairness to Grandfather, while he was in South Africa he had broken the World Land Speed Record as it stood when he left England by 12 mph and set new records for five miles and five kilometres. But people were not interested, as by then Henry Seagrave had done more than 231 mph at Daytona.

Seagrave was acclaimed for what he had done and the King conferred a knighthood on him. Grandfather's cable to him from South Africa conveyed congratulations, yet by its cryptic nature also betrayed some of his feelings: 'Damn good show, Campbell.' Sir Henry Seagrave, as he then was, turned his attention from land to water, and determined to win the World Water Speed Record. He succeeded, and then in trying to take the figure over 100 mph his speedboat, *Miss England II*, flew into the air on Lake Windermere, crashed back to the surface and sank. Sir Henry died a couple of hours later. At that time Grandfather, as far as I know, had never considered tackling the World Water Speed Record.

If Grandfather ever had a quiet period in his life it was after his return from South Africa, though a lull for him was more tempestuous than a routine day for most people. He concentrated for a time on his Bugatti agency, and it was as a car salesman that he had his next brush with death. A customer complained to him at Brooklands that the model which he had bought from Grandfather would not do the expected 100 mph. While the conversation was going on, Leo, on behalf of Malcolm, was beginning to have a look at the engine. Without warning, Grandfather lost his patience with the customer and declared that he would show him whether the car would do 100 mph or not. He leapt into the car, commanding Leo to join him. Leo responded so promptly to Grandfather's fiery command that he forgot to fasten the bonnet securely. At over 80 mph it lifted off and, as it came back over the car, knocked Malcolm out cold. Leo saved the day by taking the wheel and leaning across to switch off the ignition. He probably saved both their lives by doing so, but Malcolm's wrath with the customer and embarrassment that he had been made to look a fool meant that Leo had to take the blame for the whole affair.

Such an energetic and ambitious man as Malcolm Campbell could not be diverted from his ultimate goal for very long. Early in 1931 he went to Daytona Beach again and, somewhat unusually, things went well. Bluebird had been rebuilt under the guidance of an up and coming designer, Red Railton, and in February that year Grandfather became the first man to exceed four miles a minute. This was the triumph for which Malcolm had worked and waited for so long. In Washington he was received by President Hoover, and all the way across the Atlantic on board the liner *Mauretania* he and the team were feted as national heroes. At Southampton, when the *Mauretania* docked, the quayside was lined with thousands of cheering people. Grandfather and his party boarded a private train – the Bluebird Special – for London. A reception in Grandfather's honour had been prepared at Westminster City Hall, and the knighthood which he prized still more than the honour of being the fastest man in the world soon followed. Sadly for him, Dad was in bed at school with flu when all this was happening, but my Aunty Jean was present at Westminster Hall, to see all the famous people who were there and to hear the speeches which were made, though as a child the thing which she remembered most clearly, when she told my father about it, was being frightened by all the photographers' flash-bulbs going off.

Sir Malcolm had never been lacking in confidence, but now that confidence was overwhelming. He was certain that Bluebird had still more to give and he wanted to win the Wakefield Trophy again, although no other contenders for the record were on the scene. Lord Wakefield had offered his trophy in 1928 to any driver who broke the existing World Land Speed Record and with it went a prize of £10,000.

The 1932 visit to Daytona had something of the atmosphere of a lap of honour about it, though it still demanded all the dedication and discipline which goes with high-speed driving. Sir Malcolm increased the World Record to 253.9 mph, broke his own record for five miles, and also five and ten kilometres, and then, as a bonus, set a new class record for one of those wonderful little cars of the time, the Austin Seven, by taking one up to 94 mph.

If I have given you the impression that my grandfather was a man with one interest and one interest alone, I have misled you. Had that been so he would have been a bore. It is true that he was single-minded about speed and never doubted his ability to be the best in the world, nor did he compromise in any way the high standards he set for those who worked for him. But he also enjoyed horse riding, was keen on yachting and fishing, bred dogs and found great pleasure in travelling. His faults were those of a man who was over-energetic, over-demanding, and self-opinionated, according to those who knew him. Though Douglas Young-James in his book *Donald Campbell – an Informal Autobiography* describes Grandfather as being 'modest and unassuming', it is not an impression which has otherwise been passed on to me.

By the time he reached the height of his fame he had become the Motoring Correspondent of the *Daily Mail* and also *The Field*. This and his business income, with what he inherited from his father, made him a man of very considerable means, yet he was known for his meanness unless the money was being spent on a record attempt. In Reigate, where he did most of his shopping, he would always argue about the price of any item which he wanted to buy. His reputation was such that the shopkeepers would tell him that something cost more than they were charging to other customers, so that in response to his bargaining they could reduce it to its normal price. The result was that his parsimonious nature was satisfied and they avoided making a loss on the sale.

Leo Villa had the job of looking after the team's expenses on some of the overseas trips and describes in his book how he had to account for every penny. If he included a tip for a taxi-driver Grandfather would say, 'If you want to impress someone with your generosity, do it with your own money.'

It is said, though I cannot vouch for the truth of the story, that when Grandfather received his knighthood, the King, after saying 'Arise, Sir Malcolm', leaned forward and asked with some concern, 'Why do you do it?' Grandfather, thinking of the Wakefield Trophy, is said to have replied, 'Can you think of a better way of making £10,000, Your Majesty?' It is said of Scotsmen that they keep the Sabbath and anything they can get for nothing, and Malcolm lived up to it. The fact that he paid for almost everything he did in racing and record breaking out of his own pocket may help to explain this. This was partly from choice, but also because the concept of sponsorship was not as developed then as it is now. Many of my father's efforts were backed by commerce or industry, and I have been almost completely dependent on the support of sponsors. The rights and wrongs of this we could argue forever, but I know how grateful I have been not only that someone else is picking up the bill, but that they are providing the emotional back-up which anyone in such an individualistic sport as ours needs.

Rolls Royce did not sponsor Grandfather but they were more closely associated with his assault on the 300 mph barrier than they had been previously. A 2,500 hp R-type supercharged engine which they provided on very favourable terms meant that another rebuild was required for Bluebird. It was a rush for the body designers Railton and Vickers to get the work completed in time for the 1934 season, and when she reached Daytona countless snags cropped up. At such high speeds the problems were not now so much mechanical as aerodynamic. Grandfather established a new world record but it was 20 mph short of the 300 mark which he had set as his target, and that was not good enough for him.

Such was Grandfather's impact on the Americans that the State of Utah invited him to have a go at the record at Salt Lake City. The salt there is very hard, with crystals so sharp that they would cut your skin if you fell on the surface, yet, as Leo and two Dunlop specialists discovered on a preliminary look at the lake, they were much kinder to tyres. One factor in this is that when a car's speed approaches 300 mph, instead of a tyre having a rounded surface in contact with the ground, centrifugal force pulls it out into a V-shape and even if there is a blow-out it will continue to support the car. A front tyre did burst on Malcolm's first run at Salt Lake City, but he was unaware of it until his speed dropped below 200 mph.

This was to be Grandfather's last World Land Speed Record, and there has always seemed to me to be something slightly romantic about the fact that it was also the first in which Daddy was actively involved. He was fourteen, and Leo Villa recalls seeing father and son chatting briefly after Bluebird had been pushed out onto the blinding whiteness of the Salt Lake and before she roared away into the shimmering heat and blinding dazzle.

Dad jumped into a support car which Leo was driving, and they raced after Bluebird at 90 mph. As they approached the end of the course they could see that all was not well. As they neared the stationary Bluebird, my father opened the door of the car and jumped out to go and see what was happening, not realising that they were still doing 20 mph. He fell and hurt himself quite badly, but he learned that in such an environment it is easy to misjudge speed as there are no landmarks by which to measure it.

Bluebird had burst a tyre which by then was on fire, Grandfather had almost been choked and the windscreen had misted over. It demanded a mammoth effort to get the car turned round in the limited time allowed. With minutes to spare she was away, and Dad and Leo were chasing behind her in the attending car. By the time they reached the starting point Grandfather was out of Bluebird. Exhausted but exhilarated he shouted, 'Donald, I've done it, I've done it!'

His claim to have passed 300 mph was based on his own reading of the instruments in Bluebird. When the timing officials returned they put the figure at 299.9. Malcolm was amazed and annoyed; he made it quite clear that he thought they were wrong and would prove them to be the following day. This was not necessary as later the officials admitted to an error and conceded that the 300 mph barrier had been breached with a new record of 301.13. Grandfather's rage could scarcely be contained. They had, he told them in the most forceful terms imaginable, robbed him of a moment of glory and satisfaction towards which he had worked for a half a lifetime. Malcolm was always intolerant of mistakes, but to think that an error in timing had deprived him of such a moment of elation infuriated him. If there could be any compensation for the edge being taken off such a high moment in his record breaking career, it came a few weeks later. He took Bluebird to Brooklands for a drive past, and found that all the 30 mph speed limit signs in the area had been changed to read 300 mph!

Grandfather was now fifty and had fewer cars than for some years. He travelled to his office in London's Piccadilly each day, but had also obtained a financial interest in Brooklands and often acted as a steward there. The family home had moved from Povey Cross to Headley Grove, a fine house which is not far from Box Hill, in Surrey. He had ambitious new workshops built and told the ever-faithful Leo Villa that from then on they were to be inventors. There was something almost schoolboyish about the announcement.

I find it sad that what he had not told Leo was that already he was having a boat built in the Isle of Wight,

with which he hoped to win the World Water Speed
Record for Britain. After all, Leo had given of himself
and sacrificed much of his home and family life in
Grandfather's quest for the World Land Speed Record.
But that, I'm afraid, was the way my grandfather did
things.

Bluebird – what other name could she bear – was
a hydroplane, and was named on Loch Lomond by
my grandmother, now Lady Campbell, in 1937. After
a tedious month of waiting Grandfather decided that
if he was going to break Gar Wood's Water Speed
Record of 124.8 mph it would have to be in more reliable weather than Scotland could provide. In much the
same way as the Land Speed Record attempts had been
thought of as an attraction which would bring visitors
to Daytona, so Locarno, on the shores of Lake Maggiore
in Switzerland, thought Grandfather and *Bluebird* would
promote tourism there. During the summer of 1937 the
city provided the whole team with accommodation and
promised that steamer services on the lake would be
suspended to allow the record attempt to take place.
Added to that, the lake was almost always calm and
the weather reliable. What was difficult was getting
Bluebird to Locarno. She was too wide to go through
the St Gotthard tunnel by rail, and the only way was
to have a special cradle built and to take her through
the Simplon Pass on an adapted lorry.

Such was the excitement in Locarno when *Bluebird*
arrived that the local Roman Catholic priest offered
to bless her. A Protestant from Scotland with certain
anti-Catholic traits though he was, Grandfather could
do no other than accept the suggestion as a token of
kindness.

The record breaking bug which had spurred him
on so much on land was now beginning to affect him
on water as well. He raised the record twice – from
124.86 to 126.33, and then to 129.5 mph – and had
plans to do better still, but he was preoccupied by

two things that summer in Switzerland. Donald had been in bed with rheumatic fever at Headley Grove for four months, and he was concerned that war in Europe was becoming unavoidable. He sent Dad to Cannes in the autumn to get away from the winter chill of England, and with additional hopes that he would improve his French. In anticipation of war he had an air-conditioned air raid shelter built at Headley Grove and tried to persuade the government to build public shelters under all London's parks, but he was ignored as a warmonger.

Next year, in 1938, he pushed the record up to 130.93 at Halwill in Switzerland, but the existing *Bluebird* had given all the speed she could, and it was time for her to be succeeded by something still more efficient. Grandfather's requirements were met by a three-pointer. This was a boat which travelled on two shoes on the outer edges of the forward part and one under the transom at the stern which reduced the surface in contact with the water and so gave more speed with less power. He took the new *Bluebird* to Coniston Water, in the Lake District. When one or two initial problems had been ironed out, on an August Saturday two weeks before the war started he set up a new record of 141.74 mph.

War brought record breaking to a halt but it was something that Malcolm was willing to forego in the cause of a greater good. Much though he enjoyed the challenge of speed and rivalry with other designers and drivers, he was a patriot first and foremost. His record breaking had been done for Britain, but in 1939 the country's way of life and sphere of influence was under threat from the forces of Nazism and no effort was too great to defend what he loved and defeat what would destroy it. All his energy and vision was directed to the war effort. As well as designing a way of converting Bedford trucks into armoured cars for use by the Home Guard he also devised a machine to test the hardness of sand on possible invasion beaches, and right through the war he was involved in special engineering projects for the government.

It was during the early forties that Grandfather was in court charged under the Offences Against the Person Act. He had been troubled by trespassers and thieves on his estate at Three Bridges, in Sussex, and so had spring guns fixed at various points around the boundary. Each was loaded with a blank cartridge and ochre powder to help identify any offender. One was triggered by an employee who was hit just above the ankle by the blank and had to have his leg amputated. The newspapers made a great deal of Grandfather's appearance in court at Lewes, but the judge fined him £5 for what he described as a technical offence and expressed sympathy with him. The injured man continued to live in his cottage on the estate rent free and Malcolm paid his wages in full.

There were many people who assumed that, when the war ended, life would resume just as it had been before the turmoil began. Malcolm realised that the war would change Britain forever, not only in relation to British influence in world affairs, but also in the way people express their support for their country's representatives in sport and the qualities they look for in their heroes. The war put a dent in the structures of privilege which had been one of the features of British life, and created more equality of opportunity. It also undermined our slightly superior approach to international competition, and allowed a self-deprecating attitude to creep in which means we do not expect to hold records or win medals. When I see the Union Jack to which my grandfather and my father strove to bring honour waved by drunken football hooligans as they smash up a channel ferry, thinking they are doing something for football or England, it makes me sad and angry that our national pride and dignity has been so completely lost.

In the short term, and at a more practical level, the war had created shortages which meant that driving fast cars or boats was a luxury whose indulgence would have to wait for better days. Even so, as soon as the war ended the newspapers began suggesting further record attempts on water and even talking of trying to recover the World Land Speed Record from John Cobb.

Grandfather married for a third time in 1945. His bride was Mrs Betty Nicory. He told the reporter at the ceremony, 'We have known each other for quite a long time and we are very happy.' The happiness was very brief, however, and after just three months Betty went to France on holiday and did not return. She told him that she realised she was 'not the kind of woman he expected he was marrying'. Just what she intended by that statement I have no idea, and at what stage she got to know André Louis, Count de la Salle, I do not know, but he was the co-respondent in their divorce, two years later.

The end of the marriage was accompanied by the maximum amount of acrimony. Betty went to live in Sloane Street, in London, in April 1947, and within a week or two the count moved in. Early one June morning, Grandfather and two enquiry agents called at the flat. Betty, Lady Campbell as she was, of course, was only partially dressed and the count was in the bathroom. At the court hearing the agents testified that they had seen one bed in the flat, with two pillows on it, which had apparently been used by two people. I find it pathetic that the bed was displayed for the court to see. Surely they knew what a double bed looked like, and what it might be used for. Neither Betty nor the count denied that they had a close association, but insisted that they had not made love to each other, and that the count slept on the settee in the lounge. Malcolm and the enquiry agents said that they saw no evidence when they called that anyone had been sleeping on the settee, but they had seen a man's suit in a wardrobe among Lady Campbell's clothes. The judge commented that he found it difficult to believe that the count and Lady Campbell had maintained so close an association without indulging in sexual intercourse, and granted Grandfather a divorce on the grounds of Betty's adultery. In love, no more than in racing, did Grandfather lose without a fight.

In what proved to be his last attempt on a record, Malcolm had the benefit of a jet-engine in *Bluebird*. The development of jet propulsion was one of the advances for which he could thank the war. When he first took *Bluebird* out at Coniston no one knew how she would respond. At first there were problems with her steering, and when these had been corrected she had a tendency at speed to bounce in the water, almost throwing Grandfather out. Added to that the weather was poor, and Malcolm was not well himself. Nonetheless, when it was suggested that Commander Du Cann, an engineer from Vospers who had built her, should drive on one of the test runs to relieve Grandfather of the strain, he was soon ready for action and putting everyone in their place as only he could.

But it was a last vain effort. The court case after one of his workers was injured at Three Bridges, the long-drawn-out divorce, his failing sight and the demands of adapting his driving to a very high-powered jet engine were all taking their toll. When *Bluebird* was loaded onto a lorry at Coniston to be taken back to Vospers for more work to be done on her it was the last time he had contact with the *Bluebird* line.

After his death Sir Miles Thomas, himself a pioneer of aviation and business entrepreneur, said, 'In all that he did Malcolm Campbell was an individualist. His death robs a world that seems in danger of becoming more and more drab of a lively, colourful figure . . . His co-operation with car manufacturers enabled the benefits of his experience at high speed to be later incorporated in production models.' While people remember Grandfather and Father for breaking records, I hope they will also see them as part of the story of the motor car which is now so important to us all.

6

The last few years of Grandfather's life were the first ones of my parents' marriage. My mother describes them as being hilarious. Dad was three years older than her and she loved his willingness to go out ahead of everyone else, his sense of fun and his complete irresponsibility. Yet he was a person of integrity who would never take advantage of anyone or play a dirty trick on them. But he was a Campbell and that means, by definition, he was restless. For example, a week after I was born Dad decided that they needed a bigger house so they moved to Lovelands Mead, at Mogador, not far from Kingswood in Surrey.

Father was also getting tired of the daily routine of travelling into London and the repetitive nature of his work in insurance. Whether he was at home or at work he seemed to have been conscious that he was the son of someone famous and found it difficult to be normal. He set out to impress people with controversial remarks or daredevil antics because he thought it was expected of him, or because he felt a family duty to be different. The Campbell name, at that stage, coloured Daddy's outlook in some ways which were detrimental and some which were advantageous. As a more mature person he grew to be a wonderful mixer in any social gathering and had the capacity completely to change the mood of a room within minutes of entering it. His restlessness about the house and his job were a stage in the development of his enviable social qualities, I believe.

With no regrets and considerable optimism Dad left

his job in the City. For a time he was a travelling salesman for a product called Ki-Gas which was an additive to make diesel engines start more readily. But he soon found this as boring as office life had been. After a week or two of uncertainty – which I suspect he did not dislike – he went into business with two brothers called Ted and Bunny Meldrum. Together they put their slender resources into a factory to manufacture power tools for use with wood. Their first product was a portable power-driven saw bench which carpenters and joiners could use on site to save time and reduce errors in cutting timber for doors, skirting boards or window frames.

Their factory, as I called it, was little more than a workshop behind an off-licence in Redhill. They employed two men to work with Ted and Bunny on production, and Father was responsible for purchasing and sales. It was at the time after the war when everything was in short supply, from steel to nuts and bolts, from electric motors to paint. They all worked very hard, and slowly – very slowly – the business began to expand.

To bring raw materials to the factory and deliver machines to customers, Dad bought a 1927 Bentley. It was characteristic of him that he would go for an eyecatching car rather than a truck for this purpose. In fact he never kept any car for more than a couple of months so it would soon be replaced in the natural course of things. The Bentley had been converted into a shooting brake by a previous owner whose pride and joy the car had clearly been. He would have been horrified to see the use to which his once prized possession was being put. On the way back to Redhill from Croydon, after a particularly successful foraging expedition for steel bars and sheeting, Dad put about half a ton of steel bars inside the car and tied almost as much steel sheet onto the roof. Going down a hill he gently put his brakes on and he had the frightening experience of seeing the sheets going over the windscreen and the bonnet and down the hill ahead of him. He had used cord instead of wire to tie on the sheets, and the sharp edges had cut through it. But he was in luck – the road and pavements were clear.

Before long my parents bought a small boat. She was an ugly tub, about 30 feet long, with an open cockpit and just one engine. They spent many happy weekends cleaning her up and then chugging up and down the Thames by Hampton Court. Soon they set out on a more ambitious excursion down the river to Tower Bridge. Neither Donald nor Daphne had any experience of boating, and Dad admitted afterwards that he was swotting up elementary manuals of seamanship *en route*. He made every mistake imaginable and a hundred more besides. Their plan was to spend the night at Cadogan Pier, near Albert Bridge. The tide was ebbing swiftly and they went northward under the bridge to take a good look at their mooring. A beautiful 40-foot yacht was there but that left plenty of room for Daphne and Daddy's boat to make fast. Well, that's how it appeared. In fact, their boat gouged into the paintwork of the yacht, leaving long weals of red undercoat as a memento of their encounter. Like a jack-in-the-box, the owner was instantly on deck giving a full-blooded nautical harangue on Father's incompetence as a seaman. Dad could not disagree, but he concealed the instruction manual.

Few sailors would consider that such a short voyage with such indifferent success would have provided enough experience to embark on a trip across the English Channel or the North Sea. My mother didn't and reacted accordingly when my father announced that they were off to Belgium. A customer in Bruges had ordered two of the firm's saw benches, and had shown some interest in becoming agents for the products. Because they'd not had a summer holiday, perhaps because he had never made this kind of journey before, and perhaps because the customer was likely to be surprised or impressed, Father decided to deliver the benches by boat.

The benches were loaded at Hampton Court and they set sail. A few miles down the river at Barking the engine failed. Donald and Daphne were below deck trying to locate the fault as the boat drifted on the tide towards two lines of river barges which were moored to a buoy. They were disturbed by a shout of 'River Police'. The tide had turned and alongside was a police launch wanting to warn them that the lines of barges were about to crunch together; their ancient bark was between them and likely to be turned into matchwood. Father said afterwards, 'A Thames barge does not look very big when viewed from London Bridge whilst it's being towed by a powerful tug, but two converging lines of them seen from the deck of our little tub showed them in a quite different perspective. Happily the river police had saved the day.'

Without further mishap the crew, the boat and the cargo reached Ostend. The Belgian customs officers' main concern was to sell them bonded stores and my parents recalled being surprised to find, in what had been an occupied country, many of the good things which had not been available in Britain since before the war.

During the two weeks or so that Mum and Dad were away I stayed with my grandmother, but I was soon to have a new home. Father was bored with Lovelands Mead and we moved with Nanny, Cook and all to Betchworth. Of course, I don't remember the house, but I believe it was a very pleasant one on the side of a hill and with a lovely view. It badly needed painting and Father decided that it would be too tedious a job to do it with brushes so he bought some sort of paint spray. Unfortunately it got out of control. The windows and patio were covered with what should have been on the woodwork of the house. For quite a while no one could see out of the French windows and the light in the house was tinted a bluish shade.

The success of the Belgian experiment in overseas selling encouraged my father to be more ambitious. The business was doing quite well but he was constantly short of money. With the Government exhorting firms to export, Daddy bought a surplus torpedo recovery vessel, *Leonis*, from the Royal Navy, converted it to carry more fuel and moved the cabins forward to leave an enlarged saloon. His idea was to tour European ports with an exhibition of the Meldrum brothers' machines, and also take along things manufactured by other light engineering companies providing they did not have a conflicting market interest. The products would be on display in the saloon which was also large enough to entertain prospective customers.

No export project could have had a more hopeful beginning. Just about everything they used on board – from knives and forks, to ship-to-shore radio – was an export sample. Making up the crew with Daphne and Donald was Edward Du Cann, who went on to have a distinguished career in the Conservative Party as Member of Parliament for Taunton, and his brother, Dick. They sailed from Westminster Pier on a May afternoon in 1948, having decided that Lisbon would be the best proving ground for the enterprise. Portugal had been neutral during the war so had an accumulation of hard currency for her businessmen to spend. After a call the next day at Southampton they set course for the Channel Islands by way of the Needles Channel.

By this time I was at nursery school, with Grandmother and my nanny again keeping an eye on me out of school hours. I suppose I had no idea what my parents were doing and probably they had little knowledge of what was happening to me. Had I been aware I think I might have been anxious.

Within two hours of leaving the Isle of Wight they were heading into a westerly gale and the boat took a tremendous hammering. There was little that they could do other than keep the engines slow ahead and the ship's head into the sea. In such rough conditions that was far from easy. They were stationary for just about eight hours, the only encouragement being an occasional glimpse of the lighthouse at Portland Bill when they were on top of one of the huge waves.

Only my mother escaped being violently seasick. She laughs now to think of Dad, entrepreneur and adventurer, laid low in the cabin incapable of controlling the basic functions of his digestive system, and Edward Du Cann, with a proud wartime record in coastal forces, decidedly green and bilious, and she – the only woman present – at the helm and in full control.

Daddy recounted the incident from a different point of view. He said that at the height of it all Edward was overcome when he was at the wheel and calmly turned round and said, 'Donald, please be so kind as to take the helm,' and then walked calmly to the portside of the wheel house and equally calmly parted company with his dinner. Father claimed much less gentlemanly dignity. The moment came much more violently and all he could do was shout, 'Quick!' and get to the side just in the nick of time.

The remainder of the journey was no less eventful. One gale followed another, the engines were not as reliable as they might have been and they were constantly wondering where they could obtain their next supply of fuel. Edward Du Cann's holiday time was running out and he needed to be in Madrid to get a flight back to London to resume work, so they made an unscheduled stop at Gijon, in northern Spain. The journey from there to the Spanish capital without any Spanish currency or visa was a test of his ingenuity, particularly when he was stopped by a Civil Guard who began to produce a pair of handcuffs.

Without Edward's experience to guide him, the Admiralty charts were a mystery to Father and the local habit of fishing at night without any riding lights made navigation after dark almost impossible.

One night they tied up in a little fishing harbour at Luarca. The village was celebrating some sort of fiesta and it seemed to Daddy to be good public relations for them to join the festivities and, accordingly, he fired a rocket flare into the night sky which brought forth roars of applause from the crowd on the quayside. That was encouragement enough, so he fired a series of coloured flares in support of the firework display which was going on. Unfortunately one of them drifted in the breeze and landed on the deck of a new fishing smack which was being built nearby. It smouldered, then flamed, a major fire was only just avoided, and the local Civil Guard felt it his duty to pay a call on the British visitors. He was persuaded not to make an arrest only after he had imbibed the better part of a bottle of whisky.

It was a relief to both Daphne and Donald to reach Oporto. Supplies and food were running dangerously low, and the local chandler welcomed them with his own hospitality. The evening they spent with him and the captains of visiting Danish and Norwegian ships was memorable for its linguistic difficulties. Only the chandler understood anyone else's language, and his English was of the pidgin variety. Voicing their thanks as they left, Daddy explained that they had to continue their voyage promptly the next day, to which the chandler replied, 'Oh good, you stay, I arrange tour for you.' There was no escaping, but at least it did mean that they saw his new house. They never forgot how he stood on the landing and explained, 'This floor for me and my family, the top for the servants and my mother-in-law.' Leg-puller that he was, Dad didn't allow Daphne to forget the place of a mother-in-law in Portugal.

Lisbon proved to be all that Dad had hoped for. As well as taking orders for many of the items they were carrying, there were enquiries for a host of other items ranging from aircraft to tankers. Socially the place was fascinating. They met ex-King Umberto of Italy, and Don Juan, heir to the Spanish throne and his wife, Donna Maria. The place was full of demobbed Kings and

Queens. King Umberto gave my parents two beautiful silver mugs inscribed with his family crest.

After several weeks Donald flew back to London to see what chance there was of meeting the demands he found for British plant and equipment. He phoned Grandfather and arranged to meet him for lunch at the Royal Thames Yacht Club, in Knightsbridge. Daddy was distressed to see how he shuffled up the grand staircase holding tightly to the banister all the way, and concluded that his sight had deteriorated even more quickly than he had expected. But then as Dad was about to put a piece of trout into his mouth Grandfather exclaimed, 'Look out, old boy, it's got a bone in it.' It was a sledgehammer blow for Dad as that moment he realised that the trouble was not with Malcolm's eyes, but with his spirit. He was depressed by the protracted divorce case and his inability to get *Bluebird* performing as well as she should have done with a jet engine. They talked for a long time over coffee as Daddy was very reluctant to leave the old man.

On the brighter side, the business was doing well. Ted and Bunny Meldrum had pushed production of the saw benches up to sixty a week, and other items of equipment which were under development were coming along well. They had moved the whole operation from the workshop in Redhill to a new factory at Horley, a few miles south.

In Lisbon, Daphne, with Dick Du Cann, had been smartening up the boat, and Dad returned to find her all spick and span after the rigours of the voyage. It did not take Father long to firm up the business deals which he had been negotiating. The day before they were to leave for home he received a very good offer for the boat and had no hesitation in accepting it as he would show a good profit. A condition of sale was that she should be delivered to Gibraltar, but as that was within two days' sailing it presented no problem. Donald topped her up with fuel and while he was doing so spotted a leak from a connection in a fuel pipe. Back at his mooring buoy he set about repairing it, but needed a second pair of hands so shouted for Dick to come and help. Fortunately, as things turned out, he didn't hear so Daddy climbed up into the wheelhouse to call again. He had scarcely got there when there was a tremendous explosion and he was blown out through the companionway, and hit the rails as though he had been propelled by a seven-league boot.

Father and Dick looked at one another, stunned. There was a gaping hole in the engine-room roof, in the saloon the carpet was in waves as though it were part of a rough sea, the furniture was at all manner of crazy angles, the galley bulkhead was bulging outwards, the companion-way jammed. They grabbed the hand extinguishers and dashed on deck. Daddy rushed into the wheelhouse but was driven back by the dense black smoke coming from the engine room. The heat and the fumes were becoming more intense, and in the middle of it all there was an ominous red glow. The extinguishers were empty and Dad recalls throwing an empty one at the growing blaze as though in some way it might stop it.

A large ship steaming down the Tagus began blowing rapid blasts on her siren, and Dad cursed her for not coming to their assistance. It meant little to him in the crisis of the moment that she was flying a red pennant, indicating that she was carrying petrol. Suddenly the jerry can containing petrol for the dinghy went off like a rocket, shooting 200 feet into the air and bursting like an anti-aircraft shell with an angry orange-red flame.

Dick said he would get the dinghy and disappeared into the smoke. Seconds later, Father says he froze to the deck in despair, fearing that Dick could have fallen into the inferno. To his great relief Dick appeared in a few minutes paddling through the smoke. Scarcely had he said that he would come on board to see what they could salvage, than there was another whizz bang as three signal rockets exploded in the wheelhouse and went shooting out through the door. Knowing that all their clothes and most of their possessions were in the cabin ready for their departure the next morning, Dad was eager to save what he could. He took a final leap down the forehatch and rushed through into the main cabin. Flames were licking around the bulkhead, and the bedclothes were already burning. He grabbed what he could in the intense heat and smoke, and as he did so more signal rockets were detonating just above his head. With a mammoth leap he cleared the forehatch, and at once took a flying stride into the dinghy in the water six feet below.

Dick at once began to paddle away, and Father for the first time was able to see what he had salvaged: a dinner jacket, a coat and a hairbrush. Once they were out of range of danger, they sat and helplessly watched their precious boat burn. The fire fighting tugs did their best but *Leonis* was only a hulk to be towed away to the yacht-basin later.

There was a cool welcome for the two of them when they entered the foyer of the smart hotel in Cascais where they were staying. They understood why when they caught a glimpse of themselves in the mirror. They looked like a couple of shipwrecked mariners. Both were black with oil and smoke from head to foot, their clothes were in ribbons, they were bruised and bleeding, their hair was singed and Dick had no shoes on his feet. And between them they were carrying a dinner jacket, an overcoat and a hairbrush. Not quite the form for one of Europe's grandest hotels.

Heartbreaking though it was to lose the boat, the more immediate problem was that almost all their possessions had been on board. It was Don Juan and Donna Maria who came to the rescue. In his more comic moments my father liked dressing up, and though it was no occasion for comedy, he and Mother were profoundly grateful to be wearing clothes given them by the former King and Queen of Spain for their journey back to England.

I do not remember it, of course, but my parents came to stay with Dolly, my grandmother, with whom I had been living while they were away. She and Grandfather had separated by then. Father kept in close touch with Malcolm, saddened and concerned at the way his health had still further deteriorated since their meeting in London. Despite Grandfather's protestations that it was a waste of money, Daddy called a specialist in to see him at home, but the prognosis was not good and he died a few weeks later.

What Malcolm's death meant to my father is hard to explain. Death always means loss and separation, but because there was this mysterious Campbell bond between the two of them, it was something more. I felt it myself in the months and years after Dad's accident, and, in a measure, still do. Grandfather had been a hard man, and if feelings obeyed the laws of logic Donald could have hated his father, for he often ridiculed and humiliated his son. Yet there seemed to be something in their genes which determined that the male next to them in the line, good or bad, kind or cruel, was deserving of respect and love. Leaving the churchyard after Malcolm's funeral Father said, 'Life seems incredibly empty.' I know only too well what he meant.

My grandfather's estate was worth £175,000, the bulk of which went to Dolly, though a considerable sum was left in trust with Father and Aunty Jean able to use the interest, and then their children eventually to inherit the capital. The incredible collection of trophies and medals, which had been housed in a vast glass-fronted wall cupboard at Headley, was distributed in the most ad hoc way imaginable. The beneficiaries were gathered together in the room where the trophy cupboard was and, under the supervision of the executors, each in turn made their choice. By the time it had all been shared out each had quite a pile beside his chair. I used to ask Daddy why we didn't have very many big pieces from the collection, and he used to laugh and say, 'Your mother hated cleaning silver!'

Goldie Gardner, an old friend of Malcolm's, was at Little Gatton on the day before the auction of Grandfather's possessions, and told my father that the American driver Henry Kaiser had said that he was going to recapture the World Water Speed Record for the United States. Dad was hurt by the thought that the record towards which Grandfather had worked so remorselessly might soon become just another statistic in the record books, and after Goldie had left he paced up and down the study, sitting occasionally in Grandfather's deepest, most comfortable armchair. What had been an unthinkable fantasy was beginning to turn into an idea. What if he tried to keep the record in Britain, and in the family? It was a ridiculous thought: he had never even driven a racing car, let alone a high-speed boat.

Daddy's decision was made, and the next thing was to enlist the backing of Leo Villa. For him, preparing everything in the workshop for the auction had been a sad business, and, with Malcolm Campbell gone, at the age of forty-nine his future was uncertain. He was taken totally unawares by Father's decision, but was thrilled to be able to continue in the record breaking business. Characteristically, he thought first of Daddy, remembering that years before Grandfather had said that if ever his son thought of record breaking, Leo was to discourage him because his reactions were not quick enough. 'You're taking on a man's job if you decide to go after the record,' Leo warned him. 'Don't underestimate the difficulty of what you're trying to do. And you must appreciate that once you start this thing you're not going to be able to quit.' Dad laughed, Leo says in his book, and replied, 'Don't worry about that, old boy, I just want to push the record up a bit to keep the old flag flying.' Leo also warned him that it would cost an awful lot of money, but Dad said that would be his worry, not Leo's.

To me, all these years afterwards, it seems sad that Grandfather did not leave *Bluebird*, or at least an option of buying it, to Dad. In fact Dad had to use all his limited resources to purchase it from the executors. Perhaps it is uncharitable to say so, but it seems almost as though Malcolm was as interested in protecting his records as he was in his son's safety. But then, he could not have known how Dad would mature as a person and a driver after his death.

Both Dad and Leo were of a mind to use the well-proven piston engine rather than the jet one which had presented such difficulties to Malcolm. The choice was made for them by de Havillands, who had lent Malcolm the jet engine. They were uneasy about my father, without any experience, taking on such a monster and asked for their engine back. So *Bluebird* was reconverted to her earlier style and the Rolls Royce R37 engine installed once more, with an R39 engine as a spare. With Little Gatton not belonging to the family any more there was nowhere to keep *Bluebird*, so my parents sold their house and moved into the Reigate Hill Hotel, where there was a large shed which the proprietor allowed Father to convert into a garage and workshop.

Leo Villa had known Dad since he was a baby, but at once treated him as a boss. He says, though, that Dad disliked him calling him 'Sir' or 'Mr Campbell' – unlike Grandfather who took pride in his title – so he began to use the term 'Skipper', which he had used in conversation with Grandfather in later years. The form of address was indicative of other differences. Donald was much easier than Malcolm had ever been. He was prepared to take his jacket off and roll up his sleeves to help at any hour of the day or night, and when things went wrong he could take it with good humour rather than anger, even making an excuse for whoever had made the mistake. That does not mean, however, that he was any less of a stickler for detail. Everything he did had to be done well.

Seven months after Grandfather's death Dad was at Coniston to make his first attempt on the World Water Speed Record. The first thing that impressed everyone was how well he handled *Bluebird* despite his inexperience. After a day or two of tuition under Leo's guidance Dad told him that it was 'a piece of cake'. He was obviously loving every moment that he was in *Bluebird*'s cockpit, but it was an attempt fraught with bad luck and problems. Spares, without which he could not manage, had been sold and he had to buy them back. He had a couple of bad slides in the boat, perhaps born of over-confidence. Everything was sprayed with hot oil on one run, and – true to form – the weather was as unpredictable as ever in the Lake District.

After months of preparation in Surrey and several weeks of frustration and driving training on the lake, Daddy was ready to go. Leo was less sure and tried to dissuade him, but he recognised the Campbell doggedness and knew it was no good. With the lake clear and the timekeepers in position *Bluebird* was towed out to the centre of Coniston Water. Full of apprehension, Leo briefed Father, and watched *Bluebird* go away, the noise of her exhaust echoing around the hills. On the way south a hatch came adrift but Dad kept control of her, and on the way back there was an oil leak. But, despite all this, Dad said that by his instruments he had done over 150 mph, which was well above the record. When the timekeepers returned they confirmed this and all hell broke loose as everyone there threw up their arms in celebration. Except Father, that is. He was unusually serious, and with tears in his eyes said, 'There's my old Dad's record gone, and I've taken it away from him.' He called for a minute's silence in honour of Grandfather. Half an hour later the timekeepers had to announce that they had made a mistake and Father's speed was two miles an hour short of the record which Malcolm had set up before the war. Bluebird's gearbox had almost seized up so there was no thought of another attempt and, in any case, the money had run out. The dejected party set off home.

At that time apparently, my nightly ritual was to unscrew every nut and bolt of my cot, and take it to pieces. I would then go to sleep lying on the floor beside it. I gather that I had quite a temper and when I was annoyed would get hold of whatever was nearest to me, shake it as hard as I could, and go purple in the face. My resistance to food which I did not like was also forceful and effective; I used to plaster my mother and spray the room with it by using a mixture of spitting and blowing.

I am sure that I was important to my parents and I never lacked for anything, but I have no sense of warmth and love as I think back to my earlier days. They were both strong-minded people who pursued interests – sometimes together, sometimes separately – in which I could not possibly be involved as a child. So at a very early stage I had to be an individual. What I may have missed of a conventional childhood has been more than made up to me by the heritage of the Campbell family, and by a closeness to my mother which has developed in the last few years.

By this time flaws were beginning to appear in my parents' relationship. Dad had grown up in an unconventional family surrounded by cars and boats, where all the talk had been of racing and records. He saw no reason why his home life with Daphne should be any different. He was uncompromising in his determination to do better than his father had done. Matters were not helped by the fact that Daphne had a particularly tidy mind. Different interests were stored in separate compartments, and something which was started had to be finished.

The break-up of Donald and Daphne's marriage was as amicable as a divorce can ever be. I don't think my father's temperament would ever have allowed it to be otherwise. For however much he failed to appreciate Daphne's feelings and was hurt by her departure, he was never vindictive. Sadly, after the divorce was granted, the King's Proctor brought Daphne back to court again for failing to disclose her misconduct with two men, when her undefended petition was being heard. The decree was allowed to stand but it must have been a very painful experience for both of them.

7

My father had very firm opinions on many things. He believed, for example, that it was not good for the child of divorced parents to have one month with the father and the next with the mother, and so on. He knew that the cunning of childhood being what it is, before so very long one parent is being played off against the other. 'Mummy lets me do so and so,' or, 'Daddy gives me this or that,' they say, and the result is unhappiness for all three. He therefore agreed that I should be in Daphne's sole custody and that he would make a financial contribution towards my living costs and education.

Quite soon after the divorce Daphne met someone with whom she fell in love, and before long they got married. His job was in the Foreign Office and I just did not fit in. As is always likely to happen with Foreign Office staff, Daphne's new husband was posted abroad, and, naturally, she wanted to go with him. Because of the nature of his work I could not accompany them, and so Daphne found me a place at what I can only describe as a boarding-home-school for infants. It was called High Trees, and not far from Gatwick Airport, and I was a 365 days a year boarder there. It provided accommodation and a very elementary education for the small children of people who have to work abroad for a period – army officers and diplomatic personnel, for example – in situations where it would not be convenient to take a child.

I am not sure how old I was when I went there so

my recollections are not at all clear, except that I know it was as good a place to live as I had ever known. I think all of us can recall the first occasion on which we saw any quantity of our own blood spilt, and I remember running at full tilt across a room at the school one day, tripping and hitting my head against the stone fireplace. I split my forehead open and was very frightened by the sight of my own blood gushing everywhere.

At that moment I knew I was going to bleed to death. I didn't, but I still have a scar as a reminder of that fall. There was also the day when I saw a squirrel for the first time. Why it was so important to me I cannot think, this creature was running and jumping on the climbing frame in the garden which I could see from the school window. I was impressed by its speed and agility but I had no idea what it was.

I remember, too, that after I'd been there for some while, right out of the blue, I had a visitor. At once she impressed me as being a very nice lady, and so I had no hesitation in going with her when she said, 'I'm taking you home. I'm your mummy.' I did not know anything different. As far as I was concerned, from then on she was my mummy. Her name was Dorothy and she was kind. Her whole appearance had a tenderness about it, her face was warm and smiling, and most of all, her voice conveyed love in its velvet tones. Dorothy was my father's new wife, and Daddy now had custody of me.

Dad and Dorothy had been married the day before, and only after the wedding had he mentioned my existence to her. I have since found out that Dorothy grew up in a family of six in New Zealand, and a very united and happy family it had been. Having been so happy growing up herself, Dorothy just could not imagine being responsible for a child and not having her with you. 'Let's have her home,' she said, without a thought. And Dad was amazed at her eagerness to take on responsibility for me.

Her first sight of me might have tempted her to

change her mind, but it didn't. I looked like Orphan Annie, she has told me since, with the only things I possessed packed into two paper bags. The staff apologised because I had only hand-me-down clothes to wear, and when Dorothy asked to be allowed to take away my own clothes she was told that all I had was a pair of brown wellington boots, which were already in one of the paper bags. My mother had obviously not realised that, at that stage, I would be growing out of my clothes every three or four months. It was, I assume, the same for other children whose parents were overseas, so that clothes were passed on from one to another in the school. When Dorothy came to collect me I was probably wearing things which had been bought for Colonel so-and-so's children which had reached me by way of Sir such-and-such's daughter and Judge whoever-it-was's offspring.

I was, at that stage, a child of circumstance, I suppose. Anything which I was without I did not lack because my parents were neglectful, but because circumstances had torn them apart and left me isolated. I had everything which was essential to a child of that age, so I cannot be angry or resentful now.

Home for me with Daddy and Dorothy was to be a beautiful little black and white Elizabethan farm labourer's cottage called Abbots, at Leigh, just south of the main road between Dorking and Reigate. It had a big garden with lots of outbuildings, and I had my own quaint little bedroom which opened off the kitchen.

My only problem was meeting Father. Since the age of recollection I had not seen him and so I did not know him at all. From my diminutive height he seemed to be very big, his voice very strong, and I could not be sure that he was pleased to have his daughter back in his life. But Dorothy was so kind that any uncertainty I felt became unimportant. She took me to the shops and bought me some Ladybird T-shirts and some jeans, and remembers me saying, 'Are these for my very own? I'll not have to share them with anybody?' She confesses now that she was near to tears, but I did not even notice. I was so happy.

It was on that shopping trip that Dorothy made it clear that I was to call her whatever I felt happy with. 'You can call me Mummy if you want to,' she said, but at once I apparently answered, though I do not remember doing so, 'I've got a mummy and she's got long red fingernails.'

'OK,' said Dorothy, 'have it your way. Call me Dorothy, or whatever you want to.' It took me some days to get round to it, but eventually it was Mummy. I do not remember knowing at that stage that I had another mother, but there must have been something deep down in my mind which made me hesitate.

Dorothy had first met Donald when she was a student at the Royal College of Music. As Dorothy McKegg she had won a scholarship in her native New Zealand to study in London, and during the summer of 1950 she and five other New Zealand students toured the British Isles in a station-wagon. Looking for somewhere to pitch their tents for the night in the Lake District, one of the local people said, 'Oh, you've come up to see the *Bluebird* and Donald Campbell, have you?' They were all mad on music and knew nothing about sport, so the names Bluebird and Campbell meant nothing at all to them. However, if there was something they ought to see they were going to see it.

They found their way to Coniston, parked the station-wagon and walked across a field to where they could see some activity on the lake. One of the men involved came over to ask what they wanted, so the most forthcoming of the group, Ava – a big, blonde, very striking girl with a huge plait down her back – replied, 'Oh, we've come to see the man that matters.' It was Leo Villa who had come to greet the girls, and, with a chuckle, he turned round and said, 'Don, you're wanted.'

In less than twenty minutes the six of them were on

106

Bluebird. They had spun Donald the most unlikely story about having come 13,000 miles to see this amazing boat and to meet the great man who was going to beat the rest of the world with it, so they were almost part of the team straight away. Dad invited them all back to the Black Bull, where the team was staying, for dinner, and then showed them the film of my Grandfather's record breaking achievements. They also met Harry Leach, a senior member of Dad's team, who had his wife with him. Mrs Leach suggested to the girls that when their tour was complete they should call and see her and Harry in Southampton.

By the time they reached Southampton, the party of six had dwindled to two – Ava and Dorothy. The Leaches were surprised to see them on the doorstep of their home in Southampton, but no more surprised than they were when Mrs Leach said, 'Well, look who's here!' and Donald appeared. Later that day he took them both on his yacht on the Solent, and, as Dorothy told me the story, 'Everything started from there.'

Dorothy says she felt very young in her outlook and experience compared to my father. She found him to be utterly charming, completely natural and highly intelligent. He had enormous charisma and could make a woman feel very special, and he certainly did that for Dorothy. He was great fun and, in some ways, like an overgrown schoolboy. Dorothy was totally smitten by him: she had never met anyone like Donald Campbell.

Donald's divorce from Daphne was well on the way when he and Dorothy met, so when she finished at college she went to live with Donald at Abbots. By the standards of those days, she felt it was a rather daring thing to do. When the divorce was absolute they married.

Some of the happiest times Dorothy spent with Donald were on water. He had a yacht called *Irene* and very often Donald's sister, Jean, and her husband would join them for a day or longer. For some reason anything funny which happens on water seems to assume greater humour than it would on dry land, and Dorothy tells me that she has never laughed so much as during those marvellous times. And some of it was at Dad's expense. At sea they were all crammed together and everyone mucked in, but whenever they were coming into Cowes they would see Father take on the role of Skipper – he would put his cap on, have the other three out manning the fenders, and shout instructions to them in a very plummy Uppingham voice. Dorothy and Jean would be killing themselves with laughter but Dad did not mind – whatever happened, Donald Campbell was not going to make a fool of himself in Cowes harbour.

For me, Dorothy was the first lady in my life. As I became more and more at ease with her and with my home at Abbots, she took me to all the places to which a child should go. Her car was a black Ford Popular. It had little power and no speed worth speaking of, but we would chug, chug, chug up the road and I would be on my way to see Tower Bridge, visit London Zoo or spend an afternoon at the local swimming baths.

Much though I enjoyed and appreciated all that Dorothy was doing, I was not used to affection and I found it difficult to respond to her warmth. She tells the story that one day, soon after she had collected me from High Trees, I was upset about something and she said to me, 'Come and sit on my lap and we'll have a cuddle,' and I looked confused and asked, 'What's a cuddle?' 'Just come and sit on my knee,' she said, putting her arms out, and I did just that, with my body as stiff as could be and my back straight as a ramrod.

When I was just a little bit bigger, we were watching the changing of the guard outside Buckingham Palace, and Dorothy was leaving it until the very last minute to lift me up to see over the crowd as I was getting heavier. Suddenly she felt my arms around her legs, squeezing to the point where it hurt. 'What are you doing?' she asked anxiously and maybe with a slight tone of annoyance. 'I don't know,' I said, 'I just felt like it.' That appears to have been the moment when my ability to show love was unlocked. I didn't know that I had been lonely but when I had Dorothy's companionship and care I knew what I had missed. There were times, she says, when in the middle of playing with a friend at Abbots I would rush indoors just to put my arms round her and kiss her.

Dorothy was also a wonderful teller of stories. I can remember her lying beside me on the bed in my little room at Abbots keeping me enthralled. Mostly they were about the war, and she and I were the great heroines who rescued someone who was in danger, or got through with first aid or food to brave men who were trapped by the fighting. And there were the glamorous moments when a fighter pilot or a tank commander would recognise our exploits and invite us to meet his men, and when he told them what we had done they would all cheer. Where the stories came from I have no idea. Perhaps some of the incidents were based on fact, but I suspect mostly Dorothy made them up. And each night at a dramatic moment she would say, 'That's all. You go to sleep. More tomorrow night!'

I have no recollection of having such warmth in my feelings for my father at that time, and I think he found it difficult having a little girl who was a nosy parker around the place. Slowly but surely, though, Dorothy tells me, I wormed my way into his heart and, very masculine person though he was, he began to show me affection, but he was always very strict with me – and I suppose I was nervous of him.

My love of horses goes right back to the days of which I am speaking and beyond. When I was at High Trees, each Monday a group of ponies arrived in a horsebox and the older girls who were keen on riding could go out on them. Never was envy stronger than when I gazed lovingly at those beautiful beasts and longed to have one of my own. At Abbots there was a pony in the next field and I used to spend hours talking to it, stroking its nose or running my fingers through its mane. It belonged to a girl who must have been sixteen or seventeen, and I am sure she got fed up with me always hanging around whenever she came to see him. But a pony was all I wanted. Nothing else mattered. I would have slept in a stable – and did many times later on in life.

Father very cleverly exploited my love of horses. He hated me biting my nails and said that if I stopped he would pay for me to have riding lessons and buy a pony for me. What an incentive! But it was still not sufficient. I tried so very, very hard for two years until Dad admitted that I was biting my nails less than I used to and gave in. The only thing that helped me during that long struggle was the fact that the girl with the pony in the field next door let me have an occasional ride on it. I was so small, and he seemed like a carthorse, but was probably not more than fourteen hands or so. Sitting on his back gave me just the little bit of encouragement I needed.

They tell me I was the complete tomboy. Those wellies of mine were always muddy, and cuts and bruises were a daily happening. I much preferred to be climbing trees or looking to see what was going on in the workshop (when Father was out, of course) to playing with dolls or pretending to be a housewife. I tore my clothes and wore out shoes as fast as any boy would have done. My present list at birthday or Christmas always centred on cowboy and Red Indian outfits, and guns rather than the things most girls would hope for.

We had a wonderful dog called Maxie, who was the life and soul of Abbots. He was a mongrel but don't hold that against him because he was beautiful and intelligent. Dad used to tell people he was a Labradoodle, and that was just about right. He was a cross between a Labrador and a poodle. We also had a pond, and, little devil that I was, I would throw sticks into the water for Maxie to retrieve. He would leap into the stagnant pool and bring the stick back. But he would be stinking. Within minutes you would find him indoors sitting on the best carpet. 'What's that damn dog been doing in the pond?' Father would say, and I would reply as though butter wouldn't melt in my mouth, 'I don't know, Dad. He must have just gone in for a swim.'

Dad knew enough about canine behaviour to be aware that dogs do not impose upon themselves a daily fitness programme, so he found my explanation unconvincing. In fact, it had been so readily forthcoming that it increased his suspicions. 'You haven't been throwing sticks into the pond for the dog?' he asked, when it happened again. 'No, no, Daddy, of course I haven't,' I responded. 'You're sure?' he questioned. 'Absolutely positive,' I told him. He kept off the subject of Maxie and the pond for a week or so, and then without any warning said to me, 'Was that a big stick you threw into the pond for Maxie?' 'Oh no, Daddy, just a little . . .' I did not get any further as I knew he had caught me out, and I also knew that of all things he would not tolerate it was telling lies. He could forgive many faults in me, in his business colleagues, or in the people with whom he was connected in record breaking, but never could he excuse someone who failed to tell him the truth. I was not slow to learn the lesson, as on the odd occasion when he caught me out I was sent to my room and a severe spanking followed half an hour later.

During those years at Abbots I do not think we had too much money. I went to a fee-paying school but certainly not an expensive one, and it was as much because Father moved about a lot and wanted Dorothy to go with him as for any social or educational reason. I say that we were not wealthy as chicken for lunch was an exceptional treat reserved for Christmas Day and the like. And that is how it was for all but the best-off until the sixties.

Daddy had a philosophy about money which I imagine, in part at least, he had inherited from his father. He was never mean as Grandfather had been, but he wanted to stop me being careless with money. The first thing I had to remember was that money did not grow on trees, and the second that no one owed me a living. They are not bad guidelines, but the way he worked them out in relation to my pocket money made them completely unappealing to me. Each week, before I could have my few shillings, whatever amount it was, I had to do something to earn it. Sometimes I would have to clean the car or sweep the patio; in the autumn I might have to pick up fallen apples or collect the leaves which had come down from the trees. I hated these jobs so much that I came to despise the idea of pocket money and chose very often to do without it if a task like that was involved. He also made me give him receipts for what I had spent since my last pocket money day, and explain why I had spent money on this rather than that, and whether I thought I had made a good decision.

As I grew older the weekly rendering of financial accounts had been extended to include an essay in which I told him everything I had been doing. I hated it, because not only was it like a school punishment which I had to do whether I had been in the wrong or not, but it also savoured of spying into the secret things of my childhood, which still today I believe should have been left for me to know about, and me alone. Never mind, I survived. I developed self-censorship so that when I was doing something I decided there and then whether it was to be covered in my weekly report.

Daddy set one standard for himself and another for me – and perhaps other people. For him it was liberal almost to the point of being libertine at times, while for me it was uncompromisingly puritanical. His great saying was 'Do as I say, and not as I do'. I could see the fallacy behind it while I was still very young, but did not dare to question it. If the truth were known, in my heart I probably felt that though there seemed something dubious about what he said, it was probably I who was wrong. Throughout my childhood I had an overwhelming respect for my father. To me, he was

God. What he said was right, and had he said, 'Gina, the most sensible thing for you to do is put your arm in the fire,' I would have done it.

While we were at Abbots we had a lot of help from Mr and Mrs Botting. Mr Botting was a splendid gardener, and his wife used to help with the kitchen and cleaning duties. They lived in a very solid country cottage set in the middle of a field, with no road passing it or leading to it. When I was preparing this book I went to see them, and they are still living in the same house and, now in their eighties, are as kind, friendly and cheerful as ever.

Albert Botting had been gardener for some years at Abbots before my father bought the house. Dad, he says, liked the garden to look colourful and tidy, but he had little or no idea of how to achieve the results he hoped for. Mr Botting speaks highly of Dad as an employer, and obviously we got on well as quite often I used to stay at their cottage at Gadbrook. They had four daughters and I was almost the fifth. In their garden they had a low fence onto which Mr Botting had fixed a saddle, and their daughter Celia – the one to whom I was closest – and I used to argue whose turn it was to ride on this 'horse'. The house was so remote that it did not have electricity or a mains water supply. The toilet was a thunder box up the garden, and instead of having a door there was just a sack hanging down to preserve your modesty. In winter it was sometimes necessary to clear the snow from the seat before sitting down.

Mr Botting remembers me as a little horror who was always wanting him to retrieve the arrows from my wild west outfit which had got stuck up a tree, or demanding to sit on top of a wheelbarrow-load of grass recently cut from the lawn as he took it to the compost heap.

Whenever I went to Gadbrook I always wanted to see Bert's ferrets. They were (as I thought) dirty, smelly creatures which he kept in a small hutch and used for catching rabbits. They were quite vicious, but he would put them into a sack, and walk around all day waiting

113

for the right moment to put one into a hole to chase the rabbits out. It all sounds very cruel, but then many of the things which are taken for granted in the country look like that to us 'townies'.

I was fascinated by the lads who came to visit the elder Botting girls. Their would-be boyfriends turned up on motorcycles, and I used to pester them until they gave me a ride on the back. Just imagine it. To me, these teenage boys were as big and strong as men and I would perch on the pillion seat with my arms wrapped around them as we bounced over the rough field. It felt as though we were doing sixty and I was always thrilled, but in fact we probably did not exceed fifteen miles an hour.

Mr and Mrs Botting remember me as a tough child. Two of the local boys were playing at Abbots one Saturday morning soon after Daddy had had the drive relaid with loose shingle, and I pushed them off their bikes. The grazes on their legs were awful, and Mrs Botting told me I was a naughty girl and asked why I had done it. Apparently I said, 'You didn't see what they did to me. It serves them right.'

Occasionally Mr Botting would stay in the house during the evening if Father and Dorothy were going to be out, and he says that during one such stay I came down completely naked, jumped onto his lap and asked, 'Do I smell nice?' I was wearing samples of every kind of perfume, powder and make-up which I could find on Dorothy's dressing table.

On one of the nights when Mr Botting was baby-sitting Dad left with the usual instruction, 'See that Gina's in bed by seven o'clock and no later.' But I liked to play in the bath, and was still there at well past seven-thirty when I heard the car returning. I leaped out of the bath, raced along the corridor to my room and into bed without drying myself or putting on my pyjamas. When he'd collected whatever it was he had forgotten, Dad glanced in and said to Dorothy, 'She's fast asleep.'

114

My more memorable baths in those days were at Mr and Mrs Botting's home. In winter, their daughter Celia and I would be put into a tin bath together in front of their kitchen fire, and when the weather was hot we would have our bath in the garden and run around naked until we were dry.

It was typical of Dad's kindness and sense of fun that when Mr and Mrs Botting's daughter, Inez, was getting married he said that he would drive her to and from the church. He hired a chauffeur's uniform and cap, but a day or two before the wedding developed chicken pox. Mr Botting was very worried and on the Thursday evening when he had finished work went in to see Dad and ask whether he should make other arrangements. Dad was furiously indignant. 'What do you mean, Bert?' he raged, 'I thought you'd worked for me long enough to know that my word is my bond. I shall drive that girl to and from the church even if I have to get up from my bed to do it.' And that's what he did, but I wonder how many of the guests shared the joke.

Not only did Mr and Mrs Botting stay with me when Dad and Dorothy were out, but Dad would never allow Maxie to be in the house alone. In those circumstances, as soon as they were out of the door, Maxie would go straight up to Dad's bed and stretch out on it with his head on the pillow. When they returned he would hear the car coming when it was still half a mile away and be at the door to meet them. Dad thought more of that dog than he did of himself, and there's a lovely picture of Maxie sitting upright in a chair at Abbots, with Father's pipe in his mouth.

Daddy took Maxie to Rules, the smart London restaurant, one evening, and the waiter told him that he could not bring the dog in. 'Why not?' Father asked. 'This is only for diners, sir,' came the answer. Dad pulled up a chair beside him, sat Maxie on it, fixed the serviette in his collar and ordered him a three-course meal. I was dying of embarrassment, but this was only the first of a number of occasions when Father entertained Maxie in style at Rules, and he became something of a mascot among the staff there. The only time I saw Daddy cry was when Maxie was put to sleep.

For four or five years Dorothy was in every way a mother to me, but as time went by I sensed that she was not always happy. As far as I can remember, she and Father never had arguments in front of me but there were occasions when I heard voices raised, and when they were very cool towards each other for several days. The climax came when I met Dorothy at the front door one day and she was dressed to go, her cases and bags with her. With considerable emotion, but without saying anything critical of Dad as far as I recall, she explained that she had to go and live somewhere else. I could not understand why and passionately pleaded with her to stay. We were both in tears, and in my final effort to persuade her I said I would give her my set of specially minted Coronation coins. They had been my most treasured possession since they were given to me when the Queen was crowned in 1953. Looking back on it, I suppose it was pathetic, but it shows just how much Dorothy had come to mean to me. She did, in fact, change her mind and stay but I am sure my Coronation money had nothing to do with it. She knew that being married to Donald Campbell carried with it a responsibility for Gina Campbell, and my pleading made her have one more go at making a life with a man whom she loved but found impossible to live with. I like to think that I can take credit for keeping them together for just a little longer.

One of the things Dorothy had to learn to endure was having a jet engine in the garage. It was a spare for *Bluebird* and I remember thinking how frighteningly big it seemed the day it arrived. It had to be tethered to the garage floor with chains, and, as his party piece, Dad would occasionally start it. It made such a noise that he would always warn the local police, and then make sure that I was not in my bedroom – which was next to the garage – and have everyone else leave the house. If any of the men were working on the flower beds they would find a job to do somewhere else. Then suddenly, with an incredible roar, flames would shoot out halfway up the drive. It was deafening. You'll have some idea of what I mean if you have ever been at an airport when a pilot has given a plane's engines full throttle just before take-off. And that was happening in our garage!

I think I must have been naive or gullible as a child; certainly I was unquestioning. It never occurred to me that there was anything unusual about my father having a jet engine in the garage. Other girls' dads played rugby, belonged to the Rotary club, or collected stamps. Mine kept a jet engine in the garage! My life had really been very sheltered, but I think this ability to accept things as they came along helped me a great deal. My Aunty Jean used to feel sorry for me and say, 'Poor little Gina, she's had such an up and down life.' Seen from other people's point of view it must have looked like that. But not to me. If things around you have always been changing, then life, as far as you are concerned, is always about change, and you never miss the constancy which you have never had. I feel that I had a wonderful childhood and would not change it for anyone else's. To me it would seem much more unsettling for the blissful Mr and Mrs Average to provide a happy life for their children until they are fourteen or fifteen and then split up and go their separate ways. I was always with my father; it was just that his partners changed from time to time.

Though slowly I did become part of his life, Father's attitude to me was always austere. We were once at the table at Sunday lunchtime and I complained about what Dorothy served me. Father didn't say a word; he just got up, took my meal away and put it onto the floor for Maxie. In one gulp it was gone. He then went to

117

the cupboard – still without saying anything – took out a tin of dog food and very deliberately opened it. It was a very cheap brand, I remember, and gradually it dawned on me what he was doing. His silence made me tremble inside. He picked up my plate from the floor and without any hurry put the dog food onto it. 'Now eat that,' he said, 'and don't leave this table until you do.' I sat there in utter amazement and Dorothy was horrified. Tears welled up in my eyes but I was determined not to cry as I knew this was my will against his. We faced each other for an hour or more. Very coolly he would look at his watch from time to time until eventually there was no way out. It was not until he saw me take a forkload of dog food and lift it towards my mouth that he took the plate away and gave me some fruit to make up for the lunch I had missed. Even today, I still eat whatever is put in front of me.

I'm sure that I had no idea what Daddy did for a living at that stage. I know that sometimes he and Dorothy would be away for several weeks, and I suppose now that those were the times when he was making an attempt on the record. They never allowed the impression to get through to me that anything out of the ordinary was going on. Dorothy admits now to the anxieties she felt for his safety at the time, but with a kind of kiwi approach to things she says, 'I knew a man had got to do what he'd got to do.' To keep expenses down she was always very busy when a record attempt was on, caring for the rented house in which the team would be living and preparing meals. What looked very glamorous to outsiders was sheer hard work for all of them.

Dorothy was at home on her own one evening watching television, when she had that feeling which lots of us have had: 'I could do that as well as she can,' she said, of whoever was on the screen. She had better grounds for saying this than most of us, as she had been acting and singing in New Zealand since she was a child, and

118

she had her Royal College of Music training behind her too. With my grandmother's encouragement, she wrote to the BBC and an audition followed. She turned up dressed like a model in a black suit and mink coat, and the producer decided that she was just a rich bitch wanting to try her wings. With surprise, he said after she had taken her turn, 'You *can* sing.' 'That's what I came here for,' Dorothy replied.

The outcome was that Dorothy became the hostess of a revue called *Quite Contrary*, which was broadcast live once a week between eight and nine in the evening. The show consisted of contrasting turns from all over the world.

Dorothy can scarcely credit the coincidence that half an hour before her first show on 16 November 1955 she received a telegram from Dad saying that he had set a new World Water Speed Record of 216.2 mph on Lake Mead, in the USA. The producer was quick to spot the potential of the telegram's arrival and had it presented to Dorothy again on stage during the show. It brought everything to a standstill. The orchestra stood and joined the audience in applauding Dad, and all the other artistes on the show came on from the wings. The impact was even greater because until then no one had known that this 'rich bitch' was the wife of Donald Campbell. Few people can have begun a television career more dramatically.

Never have I received such an acclamation because I am Donald Campbell's daughter. Most of the time, though, I was aware that because he was famous people have expected me to be different from everyone else. At times it was an advantage, but more often not. At school, for example, some girls were cool towards me because of who Dad was, while others just hung on to me for the same reason. Teachers tended to go out of their way to indicate that they were not showing me any favouritism, and I got a ruler across my knuckles and was made to stand outside the Headmistress's office more often than most. I just yearned, proud though I was of Dad, to be accepted for what I was myself and for people to recognise that I had virtues and faults the same as any other child.

Sadly, things began to go really wrong for Dorothy after Father attained that record. He was so badly bitten by the speed bug that he just wanted to go on and on, and anything else – Dorothy included – was an obstacle and a nuisance. Perhaps if she had been a little older she would have known how to handle him, or maybe they should never have married in the first place. The break-up was very painful for both of them. Father would have been content to continue the marriage, each going their own way and having their activities and affairs as they wished. But this was not for Dorothy. She loved him and anything less than a shared life would have been a farce to her.

Dorothy has said little over the years about Donald but she has told me that she has no regrets at all about the five years she spent with him, and feels no malice towards his memory. He was always going to be his own man, and she never found this determined, independent quality in any way annoying. 'He was,' she says, 'a wonderful husband, but he was constantly restless to get on with his record breaking.' In the end, she felt that it was not only best for her, but for him and me as well, that she went. Father just needed to be the record holder for his country, for himself and for Grandfather.

There was something almost eerie about the way in which Malcolm dominated Donald and Dorothy's marriage. As soon as they met, Father had shown Dorothy and her friends a newsreel of him driving, and Donald was always trying to emulate him. The impact was such that Dorothy says she came to hate even the mention of his name. She also claims that I have a similar obsession with my father, and that he is still the unseen motivator in so much that I do.

Father was very clever in the way he told me that

Dorothy had gone. He knew how fond of her I was, and that it would be difficult, so he came to see me at school to say that we would be going to America the following day. Naturally, I was over the moon with excitement and, of course, asked whether Dorothy would be coming. 'No,' Dad said, 'Dorothy has decided to go home to her family in New Zealand and will not be returning to Abbots.' I was very upset, but I have to confess that the thought of going to the United States soon took over in my mind, and within weeks I had forgotten Dorothy. Looking back now, I find it difficult to understand how I could have been so fickle.

My second home during this period of turmoil was the Seven Stars at Leigh, in Surrey. I was so much part of the family there that I called Father's friend who owned it Uncle Nev. I stayed there so often when Father and Dorothy were away that I carved out for myself a role helping to prepare bar snacks and washing up. The Seven Stars was perhaps Father's favourite pub. He used to meet Norman Tebbitt, who was then an airline pilot and went on to be a prominent member of Margaret Thatcher's cabinet, for a drink there from time to time.

With Dorothy's departure a very happy phase in my life came to an end. It was not until 1984 – more than twenty-five years later – that my phone rang and a voice with a New Zealand accent said, 'Hello Gina, this is Doro . . .' She did not need to say any more. We said all the usual things about how we were and where we had been. Dorothy was in London and the following day we met for lunch. It was as if the intervening years had never been. We just picked up where we had finished although I was so young when she left.

8

Courage is not being unaware of danger, but being
aware of it and doing what puts you at risk just the same.
Malcolm left Donald little of his wealth but a great deal
of the family's pugnacity. Knowing that Grandfather's
last attempt on the World Water Speed Record had been
unsuccessful, and that he had not learned how to use
a jet engine effectively on water, Father would have
been less than a Campbell had he not wanted to take
up where Grandfather left off. He had no experience of
high-speed driving on either water or land, but he was
well aware of the risks involved at the speeds required
to earn records. He was caught in a pincer grip between
what was needed for the honour of the country, and the
family, and what reason said he was capable of doing.
It was a frightening inheritance. That he ignored the
rational and rose to the challenge is an indication of
his courage.

Daddy's great advantage over Grandfather was that
he was a capable engineer. Whereas Grandfather had
scarcely been able to pump up a tyre, Leo and the team
had to get used to the boss working all night on the
boat or the car when it was needed. In a way in which
Grandfather had never been able to do, Father could
talk with his designers on a scientific basis rather than
just floating ideas, which had always been Malcolm's
approach to the technical side of what he was doing.

But there were few other advantages. The family
fortune which Malcolm had inherited had largely been
used up, and what remained was tied up in a trust, so

that Father was constantly having to go cap in hand to industry for backing. Fortunately firms such as Bristol Siddeley, Lucas, Dunlop and a host of others responded, but they all needed to be convinced that Dad had a reasonable chance of breaking records and was not just trading on the family name. After all, he had no form as a racing driver and for him to want to tackle world records just because he was his father's son would not have seemed very convincing. At every stage in his nineteen-year career in record breaking Father used all the charm and tenacity he possessed to persuade people to put up the money he needed, or give him help in kind.

After his first abortive attempt on the record at Coniston, when *Bluebird* had been so difficult to control and he had finished covered in oil from a leak which could have led to tragedy, he says the general opinion was, 'You're playing with old iron, Donald. Pack it in. You haven't a hope of breaking the record with *Bluebird* now but you stand a good chance of breaking your neck.' Even Leo Villa advised him to forget the idea of pushing the record higher as it was costing so much money.

The logic behind what they were saying could not have escaped such an intelligent man as Dad. But there was something deeper, an inward compulsion which drove him on. With magnificent understatement, after one of his more hazardous runs during that first Coniston attempt he said to Leo, 'This job's bloody dangerous!' But he was back again the next day.

I think Dad, more than anyone else I know in sport, had his efforts frustrated by sheer bad luck. Again and again, at vital moments, the most unlikely mechanical problems cropped up or the weather turned sour, or one of the team had a mishap or illness. Coniston, where more than half his attempts on the Water Speed Record were made, seems to have this atmosphere of misfortune about it. In case you have not been there, I should perhaps explain that there are a host of deep lakes lying in the folds among the mountains of north-west England. While the area has a rugged beauty which attracts hosts of visitors it is noted for cloudy, damp weather. Coniston Water is in the southern part of the Lake District, about seven miles from Morecambe Bay. On a bright day it can look like a mirror lying among the green fields and trees which surround it, but more often mist rolls down from the hillsides over grey water and there is something ominous about the lake. I may well say that because I know what eventually happened there, but I have the feeling that even before that I did not see Coniston as beautiful or happy.

The Lake District did its worst with weather while the *Bluebird* team were there for Father's second attempt on the world record in 1950. When one of the party put his head around Dad's door one evening and said that Connie Robinson, the owner of the Black Bull Hotel where they were staying, would like everyone down for dinner as soon as possible as the water level was rising in the dining room, Father put it down to his over-indulgence in pre-dinner drinks. Without any urgency he made his way downstairs and found out how right the message had been. He knew only too well how much rain had fallen during an annoying week, and the climax had been a thunderstorm earlier that day. The waitress, a local girl called Alice, was wearing wellington boots to serve customers as there was three inches of water covering the dining room floor. A stream beside the hotel had burst its banks, causing the flood. As soon as dinner was over – which was not very long in view of the circumstances – everyone mucked in together to help Connie Robinson deal with the floodwater. The Black Bull had become second home to all the team so they were eager to help.

Before the job was complete there was a telephone call from the local police saying the level of the lake was rising and a policeman on patrol thought that the boat and boathouse were in danger. With Leo and Reg

124

Whiteman, Dad set off immediately to see that *Bluebird* and all the equipment were safe. It was a pitch black night, rain was pelting down, the wind roaring and it seemed that boulders were crashing from the hillsides in all directions. This was Coniston at its worst. They had scarcely got into the private road leading to the boathouse when they realised the water was up to the axles of the car. As the road was unfenced and had neither banks nor hedges there was a danger that in the darkness they would drive off the edge into deeper water, so they abandoned the car and with the help of two policeman began to walk the 500 yards to where *Bluebird* was.

There was only one safe way to make progress in such conditions and that was to link arms in threes. Dad took a policeman on each arm and if either slipped into deeper water the others pulled him back. When they got to the boathouse, they could see in the light of one of the policemen's torches that the water was already lapping *Bluebird*'s hull, so at once they hauled her as far up the slipway as they could. As hastily as they were able in the darkness, they collected the gear in the lower part of the building and stacked it where they hoped it would be above flood level. It was all they could do.

Only then did Father realise that Leo and Reg, who had been in the car with him, were missing. In the blinding wind and rain outside the boathouse it was impossible to see more than a foot or two, so the two policemen and Father sloshed and groped their way back to the abandoned car. Leo and Reg were huddled in the back seat. They were very wet and in the dim torchlight Dad could see they were pale-faced and miserable. Rather than follow Dad and the policemen to the boathouse, they had decided to use a fence alongside a beck as their guide. With the weight of them holding on and the force of the floodwater it had collapsed, and Reg lost his balance and fell on his face in the swirling

125

beck. In the nick of time, Leo caught him by the scruff of the neck and saved him from being swept away. By the time they had struggled back to the car they were all in.

They drove back to the Black Bull – in reverse. There was no safe way to turn round. Leo was at the wheel and my father walked alongside, shining a torch and directing him as best he could. Dad said that he was never more cold than he was at Coniston that night. The policeman who had first reported the danger to *Bluebird* had stayed at the boathouse when the others left, but after midnight phoned to say that he was by then in danger himself from the rising water. Dad called for volunteers to go and rescue him. This time, they were up to their waists in water as they struggled arm in arm along the road to the boathouse. When they got there they could just about see that the water had again reached *Bluebird*, and most of their gear – the generating set, the plugs and tools of all kinds and sizes – was submerged. One or two partly empty oil drums had floated away, never to be seen again.

Dad always made a point of being on good terms with the police and ambulance services wherever he was attempting a record, and that night he had good reason to be grateful for their help in saving *Bluebird*. The marooned policeman was taken back to the Black Bull, and with Father and his colleagues they drank the place out of rum – as a precaution against pneumonia, of course!

As it always seems to do after such a storm, the sun was shining brightly the following morning. The streets of Coniston were inches deep in mud and stones, and people whose homes had been flooded were beginning the thankless task of mopping up. *Bluebird* looked as though she had been caught by an unexpected high tide and most of the equipment was either gone or useless. Work on the record attempt had been set back weeks, but it was little compared with the job which had to

126

be done at the hotel and in the homes of the people of Coniston.

It was during this period at Coniston that my Father had one of his most revolutionary ideas about *Bluebird*. He had found it difficult to read his instruments while driving her at speed, and there was also the suspicion that her nose was tending to lift excessively when she approached 150 mph. He decided that a second pair of eyes would be useful, so a second cockpit on the starboard side was installed, in which Leo was to travel with him. To compensate for the increased weight one of the fuel tanks on the other side had to be taken out. Leo was less than keen on the suggestion and admitted to being so scared on the first trial run that he had next to no recollection of the dials, or the bow of the boat at all. It seems to me that the only possible benefit from the arrangement was that it gave Leo a close-up view of Father when he was driving which no one else ever had. His face became tense with an expression which Leo never saw at any other time. His teeth were clenched, and he had a look of grim defiant determination where usually there was a relaxed openness. Here was an intimate insight into the guts it took to defy both nature and a machine in the cause of record breaking.

After all the complications which had beset Father's efforts it was too late in the season for a serious challenge on the record. In any case, the American Stanley Sayers had exceeded Grandfather's final achievement by almost 20 mph. It was a disappointed team which went home to Surrey. The journalists, who had gone to Coniston to cover a new World Water Speed Record and had nothing to write about, were equally disillusioned. The son of the great national hero had failed to prove himself. But they were reckoning without my father's refusal to be second best.

Stanley Sayers had taken the World Record using a boat which was a prop-rider. In such a boat the propeller hub is the third point of suspension rather than the hull itself. My Father did not take long to decide that if he was to have any chance at all *Bluebird* had to be converted. The work was supervised by Lewis and Ken Norris who had been involved for some years. Now that they had set up in business in their own right as consulting engineers and designers they could be more fully committed to the project. The work was done in the workshop at the Reigate Hill Hotel, which says a great deal for the tolerance of the proprietors. Not only did they have Father living there, with dogs which tore the carpets and curtains in his room to shreds, but there was a constant din in the garage which Father had taken over. Never once did they complain, apparently.

Just how important the engineering back-up is to any racing enterprise was proved over the next few months. Without the brilliant design work of the Norris brothers, and Leo Villa's patient skill and sound judgement, my father would have achieved nothing. That is not to say that it was always a picnic. Father used to have disagreements with Ken Norris quite regularly but out of it all came a rebuilt *Bluebird* which Father hoped could sustain his challenge.

The opportunity to test that hope presented itself the following summer. Father received an invitation to take part in the Oltranza Cup races at Lake Garda, in Italy, in May 1951. Leo pointed out that *Bluebird* had been designed for record breaking and not racing, and there is a great difference. One question which had to be answered was whether *Bluebird* had a great enough fuel capacity to last the distance. And there was the not unimportant consideration that Dad had never driven in competition with other boats before. But he was undaunted, and told Leo that he might win the race and set a new record at the same time.

Lake Garda proved to be as jinxed for *Bluebird* as Coniston had been. At the beginning of the main event three attempts to start her engine failed and all twenty-four plugs had to be changed. But it was too late: the other competitors were out of sight. To be stuck on the starting line is the end for most people, but my father never knew when he was beaten. As soon as the engine fired he was away. His speed was such that Leo, travelling beside him, says he was 'nearly deaf from the noise and half dead with fear and anxiety'. Winning or setting a new record were out of the question, but the consistently high lap times proved that Dad had the cool, calculating skill which is essential in a top driver and, as a bonus, gave him the course record by a very considerable margin.

Having seen what *Bluebird* could do when she got going, the organisers of the Lake Garda event were eager for Father to stay and try for the record. He was more keen to get back home so that Lewis and Ken Norris could do more work on her. Their efforts were in vain. Later that summer on Coniston Water she hit some debris in the lake at high speed and sank. Father and Leo were not hurt, but Dad was sick that not only had he allowed Grandfather's record to slip out of British hands but now had wrecked his finest boat.

If there was a point at which Father might have given up, I suppose this was it. Apart from bills, he had little to show for two years of risks and hard work. His tried and proven boat was gone, and public interest in him was on the wane. Added to that, his lifelong friend John Cobb was killed that summer on Loch Ness when his boat disintegrated at a speed believed to have been more than 240 mph. He even went as far as to tell Leo that he could see little prospect of more record attempts until his financial position improved. Leo took a job at the light engineering works in which Father was a partner.

The fact that Grandfather had failed to master the jet engine and John Cobb had been killed driving a jet-powered boat at a speed far in excess of the World Record was, in a perverse way, an incentive to Father. Most

129

other men would have been put off by the risks involved, but Father made up his mind that when another attempt on the record was possible he would use jet propulsion. In technical terms, he knew that with a jet the maximum speed would be far greater, because the efficiency of a jet engine increases as the speed is pushed higher. The Norris brothers shared his view as a jet would have a more favourable power-to-weight ratio, and would be less complicated to install.

With the very limited resources available progress towards the birth of the new *Bluebird* was slow and painful. Calculations and drawings were discussed and revised again and again. Models were tested in wind tunnels and on water, all without anyone knowing whether the boat would have a piston or a jet engine. It was my father's persuasiveness which sorted out the problem. He went to see the director of engine research and development at the Ministry of Supply who had a couple of Beryl jets in store which he agreed to make available for *Bluebird*. Within days the first of these arrived at Abbots and the static test runs, which I mentioned earlier, followed. These were very necessary as Father, Leo, and Maurice Parfitt, who had joined them as Leo's assistant, were novices as far as jet engines were concerned. Firm decisions could then be made about the hull. It had to be as strong as a jet fighter, and while it was being built it looked more like the framework of an aeroplane than a boat.

Abbots at this stage must have been an amusing combination of advanced technology and chaotic do-it-yourself experiments. While a jet engine was housed in the garage, outdoor tests of the new *Bluebird* were going on on the duck pond. The tests involved Leo at one side of the pool, with an electric motor which drove a spool to which a strand of nylon fishing line had been attached. The line stretched to the other side where it was attached to a model of *Bluebird* which Maurice Parfitt would be holding. The point of attachment had been carefully calculated to reproduce as closely as possible the thrust of the engine and trim of the boat. My father would be in the centre of the pond, perched on top of a stepladder, with a cine camera to record the behaviour of the model as it sped across the water at 20 mph. After each experimental run the trio would troop indoors and up to the bathroom to develop the film and study it frame by frame.

For onlookers it must have been hilarious, but Dad had the capacity to ignore other people's amusement, or even use it to his advantage when he had a target in view. And once more his uncompromising ambition was to hold the World Water Speed Record. All the despair of a year or two earlier had been dissipated by a new vision.

The jet *Bluebird*'s first public appearance was at Ullswater, in the Lake District, in February 1955. As soon as Dorothy had launched her, Father was in the cockpit ready for a trial run. The new boat had never been on water before, the weather was bad and no one knew whether she was even watertight, so Leo tried to restrain Dad's buccaneering spirit, but it was to no avail. Leo describes in his book how worried he was as they towed her out to the centre of the lake. He called Father on the radio to say that the bow was low in the water and she might even be in danger of sinking, to which Father shouted back, 'Don't be such a damn fool, Leo. I know I'm not sinking because my shoes aren't even wet yet'. 'You couldn't help admiring the boy,' was Leo's comment. 'He had tremendous guts.'

Leo's admiration for Father's guts was increased still further when, during the teething problem stage, Dad asked him to take *Bluebird* for a run so that he could watch how she behaved. Leo says that he usually slept well, but not on the night before the run. Not only was he fearful for his own skin but also mindful of the cost should he wreck a boat which meant so much to Donald and had proved to be so expensive. When he was towed out to the centre of the lake he was hoping against

131

hope that the engine would not start. It did, and the acceleration was unbelievable and almost unbearable. As he sped across the lake, he was aware that Donald was shouting something to him over the radio, but his concentration was so intense that he literally could not understand or respond – and the once distant bank was approaching uncomfortably quickly.

Several more months of work were necessary before Dad and the team were absolutely sure that *Bluebird* was ready to go for the record. This gave Daddy time to develop still further what many people felt was his bluff about the water barrier. In those days newspapers were always referring to the sound barrier and its effect on aircraft. A theory had been put forward that there was a similar water barrier at about 200 mph and that it might account for the deaths of several drivers, including John Cobb. Leo Villa was thoroughly sceptical about it, and thought it was commonsense that the faster you went the more hazards you encountered. Dad always had a nose for the mysterious and accepted the suggestion sufficiently to call his book *Into the Water Barrier*, though I suspect that in his heart of hearts he regarded it as more myth than reality. He was, however, shrewd enough to know that talk of a water barrier would keep the news-papers interested, and for some while press coverage of what he was attempting had been unenthusiastic, if not cynical. Added to all the other qualities he needed to be a record breaker was that of public relations man, and he coped with this increasingly well as time went by.

It was July before *Bluebird* was ready to prove her worth. The morning of the 23rd was overcast, but the surface conditions on the lake were ideal. When the team and the timekeepers were all in position, Father was called from the hotel for what was supposed to be another day of trials. As it was the last day on which the timekeepers could be present for several weeks, it was on the cards from the start that Dad would have a go at the record. Within himself he felt like anything but

132

record breaking. He was lethargic and not particularly happy, and, most of all, his lumbago, which had started after a rugby injury at Uppingham, was playing him up particularly badly. He winced as he pulled on his light blue silk wind-proof overalls, with a built-in life jacket, and zipped them up carefully to avoid further stabs of pain.

Leo, who was in a boat stationed near the midway point of the course, recalls how he heard the distant sound of *Bluebird*'s engine start. Within seconds she was in sight. She was moving very quickly indeed, and looking a darker blue in the grey light of that particular morning than she did in the brightness of sunshine. With a roar she was past him, leaving her rooster tail of spray behind her. During the refuelling pause at the end of the first run there was time for Dad to drink a glass of orange juice and smoke a cigarette and then he had to do it all again. Back at the start, he could do little more than crawl out of the cockpit and onto the landing stage as his back had seized up and the pain was unbearable. People had lost faith in Father to the extent that there were no crowds to welcome him, and he decided not to say anything to the one or two press representatives there until a press conference in the hotel a little later. But both he and Leo knew that they had set a new world record; by how much they neither knew nor cared. Six years of disappointment had been crowned with success and in that strangely contradictory way there could be no greater sign of their joy than the two of them in tears embracing and congratulating one another.

When the timekeepers' announcement came at the press conference everyone knew that the water barrier – real or imagined – had been breached. Father had become the first man to exceed 200 mph on water, with a speed of 202.32. One of the memorable things about the press conference was the way in which Dad spoke of 'we' and never 'I'. He was then, as always, acutely aware of how much he depended on other people in his record breaking, giving all the praise to them and claiming little credit for himself. 'After all,' he said, 'I am just the man who passes water faster than anyone else in the world.'

On the day that Dad had the exhilaration of setting up that first World Water Speed Record, I was in hospital. I was a boarder at De Notta School, in Reigate, and a day or two beforehand I had swallowed a kirby grip, a hair slide which can be opened with your teeth, and then slid over a lock of hair. Unfortunately, in the dormitory one evening as I was trying to open one it slipped, caught at the back of my mouth, and I swallowed it. 'My God,' I shouted. 'I've swallowed my kirby grip,' and all the other girls laughed in disbelief. As blushes and tears came over my face, someone realised that I was not fooling and went to get Matron. Now, school matrons and I were never kindred spirits. This one was a very masculine woman with a short haircut and a domineering nature. Her immaculately starched white overall with a wide elastic belt and a large chrome clip at the front said it all. In a haughty tone, she said that I was a stupid child and could not possibly have swallowed it, and, as though to prove her point, began pulling the bedclothes apart to find it. To her further annoyance there was nothing there, and she must have had the sneaking suspicion that I might just be telling the truth.

The significance of what happened next did not come home to me until a day or two later. I assumed at the time that whenever an eight-year-old pupil swallowed a kirby grip in the dormitory at ten o'clock at night the headmistress was called from her house to supervise the rescue operation. Only gradually did I realise that these two women were panic-stricken: because of who my father was, just a word on the phone and this incident could become a story in the papers in the morning, and it would look as though girls at the school were inadequately supervised. Anonymous little me mattered to the school.

Before long an ambulance arrived and I was carried off to the hospital in Redhill. All the way there the headmistress sat opposite me and kept saying, 'You stupid child; you'll have the cane tomorrow if I prove that you're playing a prank.' I had to grin at her half an hour later when the radiologist looked at the X-Ray plate and said thoughtfully, 'Ah, there it is, beautifully lodged beside her spleen.' The headmistress's face was like thunder. I never worked out how it is that women in those schoolmarm positions can be annoyed when they think you have played a trick, and angry when they find their suspicion misplaced and that you have had an accident.

It sounds like a question in an initiative test to ask how you remove a metal hair grip from someone's insides. Smallfield Hospital, to which I was transferred after the X-Ray, devised several ingenious treatments, the most memorable of which was cotton-wool sandwiches. The theory was that the cotton wool would wrap itself around the kirby grip helping it to make a natural progression through my system without causing too much damage. It did not work that way, and when, after four days of such unorthodox efforts, I showed signs of mild lead poisoning, they decided that surgery was the only solution.

Two days after my operation, I was having some soup at lunch time when I heard the news that Dad had broken the World Water Speed Record. I whooped and jumped with glee, and I remember tomato soup spilling over the front of my nightie and feeling very hot on my tummy. By an unbelievable coincidence, Colonel Goldie Gardner, who had been a lifelong friend of my Grandfather and who had shared in the conversation at Little Gatton which led to Daddy's decision to go for the World Record, was in Smallfield Hospital at the same time as me. I remember him tottering down the ward in his dressing gown, walking stick in hand, and saying in beautifully rounded aristocratic tones, 'I've got news for you, my dear. I've just heard on the one o'clock news that your father set up a new World Water Speed Record this morning.' I can imagine the nurses having a chuckle at this gentleman in his seventies and a snippet of a girl celebrating together. He knew what it was all about but, to be honest, I don't think I appreciated how important it was at the time. The nurses helped me to compose a telegram of congratulations for Dad that afternoon, although I can't remember what I said in it, and, a day or so later, back came some chocolates and flowers from him.

Leo recalls that soon after they returned home from Ullswater, Dad invited him and his wife, Joan, to a family celebration at Abbots. During the evening he casually took them across to the barn, saying that he had something he wanted to show them. It was a brand new bright red TR2. 'It's just a small present,' Dad said, 'as a token of my appreciation for all you have done. I hope you'll accept it and enjoy it.' Leo had always thought the TR2 was the prince among sports cars.

Within a couple of months Father was invited to take *Bluebird* to Lake Mead, near Las Vegas, in the United States. It is a man-made reservoir which also provides hydro-electric power for a vast area and made possible the development of Las Vegas in what had previously been a desert. Although I did not go on this trip with Father I have since been there and had a nostalgic paddle in the lake. In many ways Lake Mead was ideal for record attempts, but wretched bad luck again took a hand. So much water was sucked into the air ducts of the engine that it flamed out again and again. At the end of one of her trial runs she had to be towed back to the slipway, and on the way slowly sank. It was one of the most devastating moments in the whole of my father's career.

American efficiency made sure that she was back on

the surface a few hours later, but she was in a sorry state. Father could never speak too highly of the way in which the US Air Force put facilities and manpower at his disposal at the Nellis air base to restore *Bluebird* to her former splendour. Four weeks after the sinking she was in good enough fettle to advance the record to 216.2 mph.

It was at Lake Mead that my father had his first thoughts about attempting the World Land Speed Record. Naturally, they were ridiculously ambitious. He had dreams of getting the record on water at Lake Mead, and then flying to the salt flats in Utah and doing the land record in the same day. With his usual realism, Leo Villa pointed out that no one had ever got the two records in one year, let alone one day, so he thought Dad was over-reaching himself. Nothing daunted, Father's targets were from then on 250 mph on water and 400 mph on land.

Back at school in England I think I was rather blasé about Father's records and his increasing fame and popularity. 'So what,' I'd say, 'your father is a doctor or an accountant and does his job, mine is an engineer who drives a fast boat and does his.' That must sound like an inverted form of vanity, but I assure you that it was not. I really had little or no conception of the magnitude of what Dad was doing.

All that began to change when I was with Dad and the team for another crack at the record at Coniston in the late summer of 1956. It was my first visit to one of the places which have become a byword in my family's story, and the first time I saw Daddy attempt a record. Young though I was, it was immediately clear that Leo Villa was the kingpin of the whole operation. To someone who has not been involved with such high performance boats and cars as the Bluebirds were, it is difficult to understand why a full-time engineer was necessary, but during that week in the Lake District I saw Leo work from morning till night every day. At times he was supervising work being done by other members of the team, but more often than not his body was in some contorted position attending to some minute detail of the engine or hull of a very sophisticated boat. Not only was he a fine engineer, to Malcolm he had been the person who absorbed all the tension which his temperament created, and to Donald he was both friend and employee, whose experience and loyalty over the years ensured a soundness of judgement which more than once saved Donald from making mistakes born of his own enthusiasm.

It was quite common in those days for children to call their parents' friends Uncle or Aunty, and Dad had encouraged me to address Leo Villa as Uncle Leo. During this week at Coniston quite unconsiously I called him 'Unc' one day, and it stuck. It became his nickname in the team, and he even signed notes 'Unc'.

The other impression which will remain with me is of *Bluebird* herself. I used to stand on the jetty by the boathouse and see her towed out onto the lake. There was a tremendous whine as the engine ignited, and the roar when it was running seemed to bounce off every hillside for miles around. At rest, she looked like a big blue whale and it seemed to be ages before anything really began to happen. Then the noise level increased still further, spray began to appear at the stern, and as she rose in the water her character changed from that of a basking whale to some sort of beautiful but aggressive bird. The jetty was well down the lake from the measured mile, so sometimes Dad would circle in front of us before putting his foot down and making a straight line past a headland and out of sight, leaving us only to enjoy the powerful sound of the Beryl engine.

On this occasion the build-up period to the record attempt was unusually short. We had arrived on a Tuesday and by the following Sunday afternoon the magic figure had been pushed up to 225.63 mph. The new record was not a particular milestone, but it was

138

important in fostering the public support which Dad had lost earlier.

There's a joyous picture of me sitting on Daddy's shoulders, with Dorothy – my stepmother – Aunty Jean and Leo beside him, and Maxie with his paws on Father's waist, just after the figures had been announced. I never knew whether Dad realised it but he set that record on my birthday, 19 September. I remember that detail because a very jolly hockey-sticks BBC reporter came up to me and said, 'Gina, Gina, what a fantastic birthday present. Could you wish for anything more?' I diminished the whole achievement – and probably put an end to his career – by answering, 'I really wanted a pony!'

I loved my father very dearly and I was proud to be in the background in his moment of success, but I felt the world of speed and the British public had taken more than they deserved of my Dad. I wanted and needed him to be around for me – just for me, alone – as Dad. I was shy of him, and I did not know how to show him that I was pleased about what he had done. The fault was probably as much mine as his, but I was not sure how I would be received if I rushed up and gave him a cuddle and a kiss in front of all those people. The uncertainty probably goes back to my childhood when I spent so much time without a close family around me.

On my first visit to America in 1958 we crossed the Atlantic on the USS *United States*, which held the blue Riband. Apart from Daddy and I, there were Leo and his wife, and a lady who was new to me called Colette. 'Speak of her as my social secretary,' Dad told me, when I asked who she was. I had no idea what a social secretary was, but over the next few years I found that it was a convenient way of describing Father's girlfriends who accompanied us from time to time. *Bluebird* was also on board as prize deck cargo.

The journey across the Atlantic was important for me as during those five days Leo taught me to swim. It was quite rough and the water in the indoor pool would be flung first to one end and then the other by the tossing of the liner. I had always been crazy about water and spent every minute that I could in the pool.

Our destination was Lake Canandaigua, to the southeast of Rochester, in New York State, not far from Lake Ontario. Neither there nor at the second choice venue, Oneida Lake, near Syracuse, did Father have any success, but for me the six months or more I spent there were some of the most formative in the whole of my growing up. We stayed at a rustic inn called Redwood Lodge, on the shore of Lake Canandaigua, and I remember that my 'home' was a chalet in the garden. The whole place was rather like the set for a twenties' western movie. The various buildings had wooden porches and verandas with rocking chairs on them. Each outside door had an extra lightweight frame door with mosquito mesh over it which clanked every time someone went in or out.

The whole set-up was managed, or perhaps owned, by a very formidable lady who had a niece of about my age with whom I played quite often. My other companions were the numerous children of one of Father's friends in the area, Howie Samuels, who was, as best I remember, a prominent local politician. I had some of the happiest times I ever remember with them; it was a great outdoor life, with plenty of room to walk and swim and ride, and weather which was incomparably good.

It was the sunshine which got me into trouble on the first day, though. Father was busy, and I was too young to realise the danger I was putting myself in by exposing my fair, freckled skin to the sun all day. With nothing more than dinky little knickers on, Susie Samuels and I spent the whole day running in and out of the water. She was used to it but when I put some clothes on later I just cried out, 'Ooh, my clothes are hurting me.' Within a few hours it was as though I was in a straitjacket. I was blistered from head to toe.

I was shivering, my tummy was upset, my eyes could not stand any light. I was a very sick girl. For a week I had to bear these third-degree burns and, with no adult really to look after me, the best I could do was to bathe myself in calamine every half hour.

Part of the appeal of Lake Canandaigua was a Bluebird Theme Park which had been set up there. Its appeal was brash and materialistic but I loved the rides at the fun fair, the candy and ice cream stalls, and the general 'come and enjoy yourself' atmosphere. There were also shops, camping sites and a yachting marina, but the novelty which really caught my imagination was the Coca-Cola machines. We did not have them in Britain in those days, and it seemed a little girl's dream that, just by having a supply of nickels or dimes with me, Coke could be on tap at any time of the day or night. It did not take long for me to observe that the machines were restocked between 9 and 9.30 each morning, and if I was there, looking dejected and annoyed, I could tell the man that I had put money in but no bottle of Coke had been supplied. He would give me one – and sometimes two. I found, after a while, that by moving quickly I could pull this fast one at several machines during his daily round. I'm sure he saw through what I was doing but regarded me as a poor little English kid who needed building up.

As I was to be in the States for some time Daddy arranged for me to go to school. In those days British children were thought to be more advanced educationally at any given age than their American counterparts. I was therefore pushed up a grade which did my ego a power of good. I was impressed by their colourful school kit. At home we had brown canvas satchels, pencils were a natural wooden colour and classroom decor was mud and deep mud, but in Canandaigua everything was colourful and the dull old satchels had been replaced by plastic briefcases in bright reds and blues. Another educational institution in the USA is the school summer

141

camp. I thoroughly enjoyed living for ten days or so in huts in a lakeside forest, eating meals in the open air, going on hikes where I saw creatures and plants which we do not have in Britain, water ski-ing and playing tennis. At some stage, most days, Dad would roar up or down the lake in *Bluebird* and I would just shrug my shoulders and mutter, 'Oh, there's Dad.' What he was doing seemed distant and irrelevant.

One near disaster which occurred while I was at Canandaigua happened when I was pretending to fish. The daughter of the proprietor of Redwood Lodge and I had watched other people fly fishing and decided to try our luck where the lawn of the Lodge ran down to the lake. We soon found that it was not as simple as it looked. Gradually I developed a skill in casting, and, showing off a bit I expect, I swung my rod and the line whirled around my head. Behind me there was the most fearful scream. My friend appeared like a mad bull with blood pouring from her ear. The hook on the end of the line was firmly embedded in it. Father was angry with me, not so much for what I had done, but because I was so unsympathetic to her. After all, if you play games like that you must expect to get hurt.

From then on it seems I spent more of my time with Howie Samuels' eight children. One advantage of big families is that if you fall out with one you can always turn to one of the others, and that is what I did. They lived in a beautiful rambling old mansion and kept several horses in their yard. We would sometimes go and pick sweetcorn from plants which towered above me, eight or ten feet high. There was a large, benevolent black lady who worked for them, and she used to prepare cinnamon sandwiches for us children to eat. It was a fabulous place – like something out of *Gone With the Wind*.

Up the road from the Samuels' there was a sort of farm where less well-off people lived. They were not exactly gypsies, but they were the wheeler-dealer type and not too particular about what they did, or how they did it, as long as it made money, I felt. I became friends with the son of a scrap metal dealer who lived there. It was not a boy/girl relationship – I was too young for that – though he may have hoped that it was going to be. We used to get off the school bus each afternoon, I would change into jeans and a T-shirt at Redwood Lodge, and go home with him, not because I wanted his company, but so that I could ride one of his father's horses.

With a group of youngsters from there – mostly older than I was – I would sometimes ride a mile or two to a place which they called Death Valley. There was something sinister about the place, I suppose, and we would sit on our horses looking over the rim of this sheer drop of several hundred feet, into a vast forested bowl below us. Hanging over the edge there was a branch of a gnarled tree with a tatty piece of frayed rope on it. Just the kind of thing you would find where children play, but I was naive enough to ask why it was there. They knew by this time they had a sucker with them, and an English sucker at that. They told me the most horrendous stories about people being hanged there, or swinging on the rope until it snapped and their bodies never being found in the near-jungle below. Each time we went it was a different tale, and each time I knew they were trying to frighten me. They succeeded! I was so unsure of myself that I would go back to Redwood and have a completely sleepless night as I lay imagining all the horrible things they said had happened, and imagining they might happen to me. Yet I always wanted to go back there again.

The place where these people lived was chaotic, with broken-down cars dumped in the fields, and pigs and chickens running hither and thither. One day when I was there, a small brown and white dog which did not belong to them ran across part of their land and the father of the family just maliciously shot it. It was not killed outright, and ran senselessly for a few moments until it tumbled into a ditch. I ran to where it was, whimpering and helpless. He came after me at once, and 'to finish him off', as he put it, shot the dog through the eye. I think this was the most barbaric thing I had ever seen. The dog was doing no harm. It was just wicked cruelty. I will not tolerate any form of cruelty to animals. They give us such pleasure and ask so little of us. I would gladly have seen that hideous man treated as he treated the dog. I found out who the dog had belonged to, took one of the man's horses and galloped off to their house to tell them what had happened. They were heartbroken, but no more than I was. I never went back to that place again.

Returning to England my father was in a somewhat morose frame of mind. He and the team had done their part as well as ever but undercurrents in the water, the presence of so many pleasure craft churning up the surface, and one or two faults with *Bluebird* herself had prevented him taking the record further. He hated not to succeed even more than most of us, and became introverted and reclusive when his lot was something less than he planned for.

However low my father's spirits sank his determination always remained. Indeed, one of the most effective ways to stir him into renewed activity was to suggest to him that he was losing heart. As though to make up for things going wrong in the States, Father set a new record at Coniston Water later in 1957 of 239.07 mph. Twelve months later he increased it by another nine miles an hour, again at Coniston. But this did not mean that it was becoming easy to break the record. In fact, the opposite was the truth. As speeds increased so the complexity of the problems and risks was multiplied, but the growing experience of Dad and the team meant that these could be coped with more quickly. By this time *Bluebird* had the tail fin that gave her the familiar profile which is to be seen in so many photographs of her.

On Christmas Eve, 1958, Dad married Tonia Bern. He

had introduced her to me in the usual accomplished way he had in potentially difficult situations. He brought her down to the school which I was by then attending in Blandford, Dorset, in an Aston Martin – impressive enough by itself. As she got out, another girl who had watched them arrive with me said, 'That's Tonia Bern with your Dad!' 'Who the hell's Tonia Bern?' I asked, which rather nullified any dramatic impression which Dad had been trying to make. Tonia was an actress, and in the hotel to which they took me for lunch played her part well and got me on her side. I was not so sure after I wrote to her saying how pleased I had been to meet her and maybe she would like to follow up our meeting by sending me some sweets occasionally. She replied saying that sweets were not good for me. What neither Tonia nor the other women to whom Father introduced me at that stage knew was that I was more experienced at weighing up potential stepmothers than they were at assessing a child who went along as part of a marriage contract. I wrote to Daddy to let him know that I thought Tonia was a bit mean, but might possibly bring me up better than someone who would pamper me.

Later on I learned that Dad had met Tonia at a bachelor party at the Embassy Club, in London, where she was taking part in the cabaret. This beautiful blonde, he said, was sitting in a glass cage, and men in the audience were provided with toy guns to fire at her. The so-called bullets had rubber suction pellets at the tip so that they stuck to the glass. Wherever they hit, the girl had to take off the nearest piece of clothing until she was naked but for a G-string. It was amazing, he said, how shaky hands became when there were only a couple of garments left. Afterwards, the girl came to have a drink at my father's table and they exchanged telephone numbers. Next morning she phoned Dad and invited him to a party that evening at the Savoy Hotel. He did not hurry to get there, and when he did was greeted by a beautiful statuesque blonde, who hardly resembled the girl at the Embassy Club the night before. Icily she said, 'You're more than an hour late.' She was Tonia Bern, and the party was to celebrate her opening at the Savoy. To make amends Father took her out for dinner a day or two afterwards, and two weeks later they were married at Caxton Hall. It was a rather quieter occasion than Dad's first marriage there had been.

Following the ceremony there was a very smart luncheon at the Savoy, and I sat next to the comedian Terry Thomas. After a bit the waiter came to our table and said, 'Madam, what would miss like off the menu?' Without a moment's hesitation I looked up at him and said, 'I think I'd like some boiled eggs, please.' 'What an excellent idea,' Terry Thomas said, 'I think I'll join the little lady.' So the two of us sat there at Tonia and Daddy's reception in the Savoy Grill eating boiled eggs!

In May 1959, Tonia had her first taste of record breaking. In conditions as good as you would ever find at Coniston, Dad set a new record of 260.33 mph. Leo Villa says in his book that she was waiting at the pier-head to greet him, looking pale and worried. She had known about Dad's courage already, but now she knew that there was a passive courage required of the concerned onlooker. Both kinds of courage were going to be needed to the full as the Bluebird car became a reality, and the World Land Speed Record the target.

9

My father had the most remarkable send-off imaginable for the first attempt he made on the World Land Speed Record. He knew well enough that he might never come back, for the history of the record is the story of the deaths of many brave men. Like so many other events in his life it was a mixture of the tragic and the comic. Many of his friends from every walk of life gathered at the Café Royal, in London, and during dinner his solicitor, Victor Mishcon, produced a new will, which had to be signed and witnessed there and then. It was, I should think, the only will ever to be witnessed by the whole of the Crazy Gang, Britain's top comedy entertainers of the time. Dad could never resist a gesture which brought fun into a situation of possible tension. The new Bluebird was the most advanced, powerful car ever built. At a press preview at the Goodwood circuit, in Sussex, in May 1960, Dad took her round the course with the brakes on to keep her speed down – and she was still doing 80 mph. Her idling speed, with no throttle at all, was 180 mph.

Bluebird had been built in Coventry by Motor Panels Ltd, under the supervision of Ken and Lewis Norris. She was known officially as the CN7 – CN standing for Campbell-Norris. The secrets of her power and speed were the Bristol Siddeley Proteus engine which developed 5,000 hp at 11,000 rpm – of the type used in the Britannia airliners – and the streamlined body and chassis which were built as one, using the stressed skin principle. She had four-wheel drive, with wheels and tyres which Dunlop had designed and made specially. As well as disc and air brakes, there was an emergency system to stop the car if these failed, and a parking brake to hold her when the engine was being started. The steering allowed only a four-degree movement in either direction, which was quite adequate on a record run, but left very little scope for manoeuvring the car at the turn-round. In length she was just over thirty feet and, with the mass of electronic equipment she carried, weighed over four tons. It gives you some idea of what a complex machine the new Bluebird was to know that the design work alone had taken 36,000 hours compared with 8,000 for the jet-propelled *Bluebird* boat.

Dad decided that the place where he had the best chance of pushing Bluebird to her full potential was on the salt flats near Salt Lake City in Utah. It was there that Grandfather had become the first man to exceed 300 mph on land twenty-five years earlier. In the intervening years much of the surface had been removed so its chemicals could be extracted and, instead of the dazzling hard white crystals which made up the surface in 1935, it had become grey, damp and much less stable.

When the trial runs began it was at once clear that Bluebird was a magnificent car, though naturally each time minor adjustments were needed. Leo Villa and Ken Norris wanted to progress slowly to learn all they could about her behaviour before putting her to the test at a really high speed. Dad was so thrilled with her that he could not wait. Before one run he told Leo and Ken that he was going to get her up to 300 mph within two miles. The two of them chased him down the course as they always did, though he was almost out of sight before they had got into their car. Suddenly, ahead of them, a cloud of salt came up and in the middle of it they saw something blue tumbling over and over. It took them what seemed like an eternity to reach Bluebird and as they neared her they passed scattered pieces of blue wreckage. The engine was still screaming away, but two of the wheels had come off. When they raised the canopy Dad was sitting there motionless, one cheek bleeding quite badly, and though he was conscious there was a totally expressionless look in his eyes. It was unthinkable that so much care had gone into designing and building this car and on its first serious run it had become a wreck. Whatever had gone wrong, from marks on the track it was clear that Bluebird had been airborne for 275 yards before bouncing four times and then sliding to a standstill.

Tonia was so new to this business that I can only imagine how she felt seeing the accident, getting to the scene, and then following the ambulance to the hospital. In fact, Dad's injuries were less than seemed likely: a fractured skull and a pierced eardrum. By the time he reached the hospital his only concern was how soon Bluebird would be ready for another attempt on the record.

Back in Britain, Sir Alfred Owen, a big industrialist in the Midlands, heard what Father had said, and responded with the offer to build another Bluebird. 'If Campbell has the guts to carry on, I'll build him another car,' he said. By November the following year the car was ready, and Daddy was fit again.

For his next attempt on the record Dad was recommended to go to Lake Eyre, about 200 miles north of Adelaide, in South Australia. Only once in a lifetime does it rain there, he was told, and for the remainder of the time the lake is an arid plain consisting of 3,000 square miles of scorched, rock-hard salt. No sooner had the decision been taken than BP Australia, who were supporting the venture, contacted him to say that rain had fallen and that he should defer his visit. In the event, it was the spring of 1963 before the expedition set off from Britain. More than eighty companies were backing the attempt in one way or another, and so, as well as the team of engineers, Dad was able to take Tonia, Leo's wife Joan, his butler and cook, and me.

I had to stay in England until my school term finished and then, when we broke up for Easter, I followed the rest of the party. I was sixteen. I remember so well how my father's secretary, Rosemary Pielow, of whom I was very fond, and who now lives in Australia, took me to Heathrow Airport armed with a ticket, a suitcase and some cash. There I met a business colleague of Dad's, whom I remember was called David. He was to travel with me on the journey. I had never met him before and he was probably very good at his job, but my immediate impression was that he was not a very responsible person. He was unshaven and dishevelled, and turned up with nothing more than a sponge bag containing his razor, and a briefcase with at most a change of underwear in it. It was not his fault, I know, but he did not have a thumb on his right hand and I remember that when I was introduced to him – typical child – I said, 'Aww . . .' and had a look of horror on my face. Remember, although I had often flown with Dad in small aircraft, this was my first trip in a large jet, and certainly the longest journey I had ever made. As someone who was rather young for my age I had hoped for a travelling companion to give me a bit of confidence, and I think Daddy too had intended that David should look after me.

On the plane he dumped his gubbins in the pocket in the seat in front of him, ordered a large whisky, and then another, and another, and flopped back into the corner of his seat to snore his head off for the next few hours. I just sat there and thought what an unattractive oaf he was. Worse still, we had an enforced stopover in San Francisco and I had to share a room with him. I was saved any maidenly embarrassment by the fact that he went out for the evening, but he got absolutely stoned, was mugged, and had all his money and his passport stolen. He arrived back to hammer on the door when

I was trying to get some sleep, and he needed me to help him get to bed. All this, after he had left his limited possessions on the plane and I had collected them and carried them for him. I was furious and indignant, and felt that I had been humiliated. I needed to blame someone but I did not know who. Whatever else, I think that journey helped me to grow up a little bit. Before we left San Francisco he had 'borrowed' all my money and cashed my travellers' cheques and blown the lot.

For the leg between San Francisco and Hawaii, I had this hungover man on one side of me flopping all over the place, and an enormous woman, who billowed out over my seat, on the other. It was six or seven hours of purgatory wedged between them, with my elbows crushed into my ribs.

Never was I more relieved to see my father than when we arrived in Sydney. My first night in Australia was to be no more peaceful, however. Right next to the Manley Hotel, where we were staying, there was a travelling circus. Sleep was difficult enough after the journey, as no one had explained to me what jet-lag was, but just outside my window the elephants were trumpeting all night. Father was no more pleased than I and at breakfast he remarked, 'If those bloody elephants want to make love, I wish they'd learn to do it quietly.' I was mystified as to how he knew they were making love, but was discreet enough not to ask.

One of my earliest social gaffes happened on this visit to Sydney. Father, Tonia and I were invited to dinner with the owners of the city's most prestigious department store. I wore my best party dress, had my hair specially done and was even allowed, under Tonia's supervision, to put on just a touch of make-up. I shall never forget the face of our hostess, Lady Lloyd Jones, when she asked me what I would like to drink before dinner, and I said, 'A whisky and soda, please.' The truth is that I was trying to do the right thing and

151

had no idea what to ask for, and the last drink I had heard of was my travelling companion's on the plane. Tonia came to my rescue saying that if that was what I wanted, I could have it. Her attitude coincided with what I know Daddy's would have been. Long before this incident, when I had wanted to smoke, he had given me a packet of cigarettes and a box of matches, and told me to go to my bedroom and see how quickly I could smoke all ten cigarettes, and then come back to tell him. I was so ill there was no question of going back to tell him. The result is that I have never smoked and am only an occasional drinker, though I do admit to a liking for champagne and white wine.

Despite the elephants and the whisky, I enjoyed Sydney. After a damp grey English winter there can be few more invigorating sights than the beaches, the sea and the sunshine of Australia. All too soon we were on our way to Melbourne where Dad had to do some public relations work in connection with the Bluebird project. I liked Melbourne because both the *Bluebird* boat and the Bluebird car had been on show there at an International Trade Fair the previous month, and everyone was interested in Dad and what he was aiming to do. Eventually we reached Brighton, a suburb of Adelaide, where Dad had rented a house near the beach, which would be our base while the Lake Eyre attempt was going on.

Dad used the months of waiting to good effect. The Australian Government had agreed to build a causeway over the salt at the edge of the lake, which was like lethal black quicksand and smelt like a sewer, to give us access to the surface. The army and the police had helped by having teams of men living under canvas at the site for weeks, who cleared the course of the thousands of outcrops of hard salt which were scattered over the surface.

When we were in Adelaide I shared a room with Dad's secretary. She was young, attractive and popular.

So popular that the room became little more than a wardrobe to her, as she seldom slept there. The sea nearby was shark-infested so for our swimming we went to a nearby pool, and in the house itself there was an excellent games room in which I played a lot of table tennis. My particular opponents in this were two 'gofers' who had joined us, both very amusing lads – David Johnson from Scotland, and Jerry Barr from somewhere south of the border – who were bumming their way round the world, for want of a better term. They had an Austin Mini with stickers from all the cities they had been in. They had worked on sheep stations, as street cleaners, bar tenders, car park attendants and so forth. Hearing that Dad was in town, they offered to do all the menial jobs which no one else cared about in return for their keep and a couple of pounds in their pocket. They proved to be invaluable, and finished up as very keen members of the team.

David, who had travelled out with me, did not survive long with Dad. They had one hell of a row after a week or so, and he left. Before that he had also fallen out with a girlfriend, who was waiting for him when he arrived in Adelaide. She was a very attractive model. In her anger, before she departed, she daubed rude things about him in lipstick on the walls and mirrors. 'You bastard' was one of the milder ones.

In an odd way, I was quite in awe of David and used patiently to run around behind him tidying up, or trying to pour oil on troubled waters. At fourteen I was realising that somewhere along the line, men and women are different. He was a lout in every way, yet in those few days I came to feel that what he needed was the feminine touch to mellow some of the ugliness of his behaviour and appearance.

Before he left home Dad had bought a Piper Apache aircraft, as we would need to commute between Adelaide and Lake Eyre every two or three weeks. My first sight of the lake was from the plane. It is a wild, vast expanse of nothing, about a third of the size of Wales. When you were on the ground, at the centre of it, where there was not a tree or a bush, there would be no clouds in the sky and no sign of water on the ground. Within seconds you would not have a clue from which direction you had come, or where you ought to go. It is so hot and the glare of the sun so strong that you naturally turn away, and at once the shoulders of your shirt are black with flies – not dozens but thousands, and once they have come they will not leave you alone. The local men walked around wearing those hats with corks hanging down in front of them. It looked ridiculous to me, but it worked. Dad carried a can of aerosol everywhere and sprayed to the right, to the left, and hard ahead as he went.

The children on the nearby sheep station had runny, swollen eyes because the flies were such a pest that the kids just mushed them in rather than brushing them away. The children looked very poor: some were Aborigines and some white, but all of them were skinny, and dressed in rags. It was almost as though we had travelled back to an earlier era and perhaps we had. It is said that the Aborigines represent the oldest civilisation in the world. Their mythology claims that in the beginning of time sweet, clear water lapped the shores of Lake Eyre. In those far-off days two of their number, Purleemil and Wimbakaboto, had a baby son in their home on the western plains. An evil man, Tirlta, was jealous of their child and their happiness, and in the darkness of night came and murdered them and went away gloating. According to the legend, this was the origin of sin in Aborigine culture, and to punish Tirlta the gods turned him to stone. The tears of the spirits turned the waters of the lake to salt and the tradition says that anyone who intrudes into its territory will be swallowed up for ever.

With his fascination for the mysterious, Father was captivated by this story. He did not believe it, I am

154

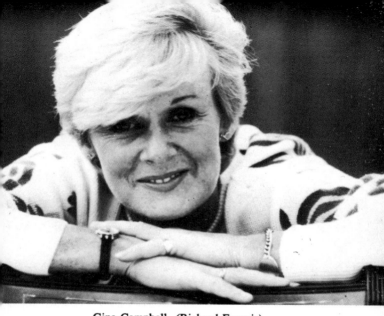

Gina Campbell. *(Richard Francis)*

Father and son, in 1933; standing beside Grandfather's Bluebird.

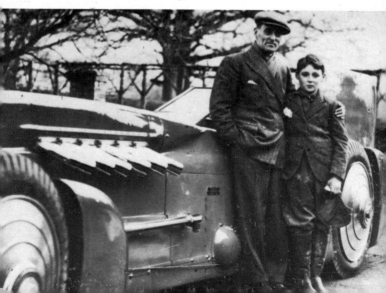

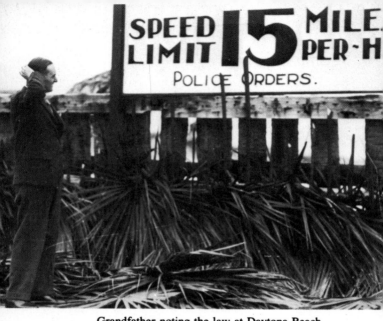

Grandfather noting the law at Daytona Beach.

Bluebird at Bonneville Salt Flats, 1935.

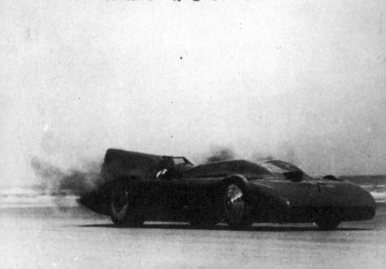

"BLUEBIRD" 276·186. M.P.H

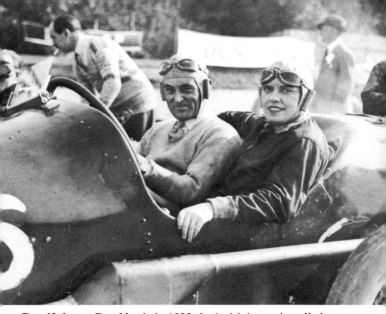

Grandfather at Brooklands in 1923; he is driving a six cylinder Indianapolis Sunbeam.

Donald at school, 1931.

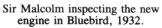

Sir Malcolm inspecting the new engine in Bluebird, 1932.

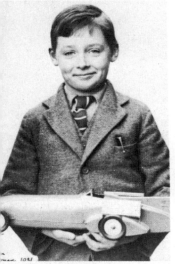

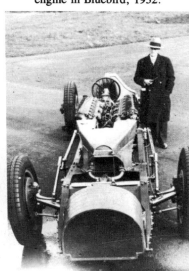

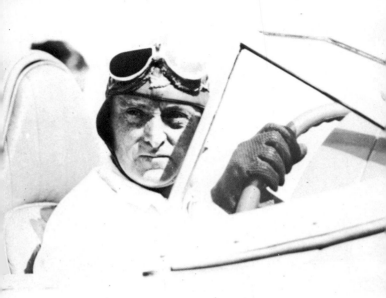

Grandfather in Bluebird.

Grandfather in the 1935 car at Bonneville Salt Flats.

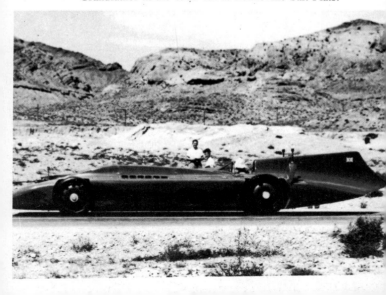

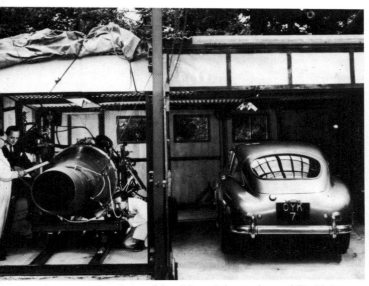

My earliest memory of record breaking. A jet engine and Daddy's Aston Martin side by side at Abbots. Leo Villa and my father discuss details of their plans while Maurice Parfitt examines the lower part of the engine.

'You're the engineer — you tell me where the hell the smoke's coming from.' Dad at Coniston in 1956.

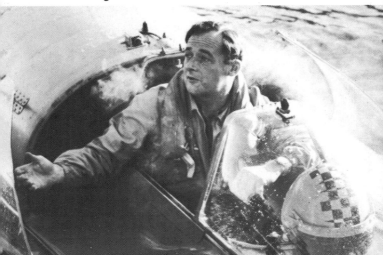

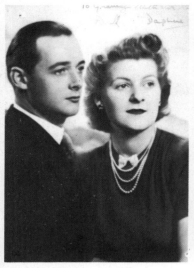

Mother and father.

Dad after setting the new
World Water Speed Record,
with Dorothy, myself, Leo
Villa and Aunty Jean. It was
my birthday.

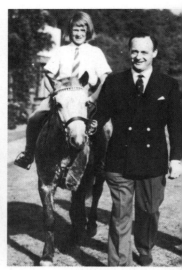

Me, Dad and Columbine, my
first pony.

Dad, me, and Mr Whoppit in
1960.

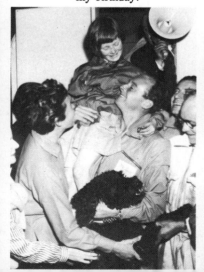

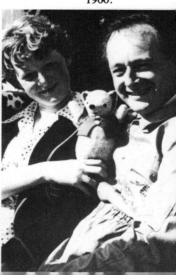

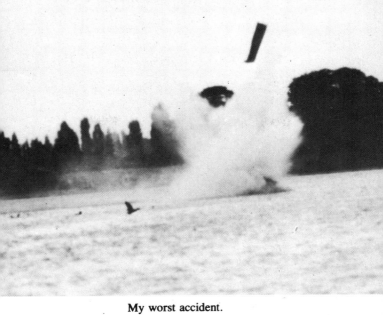

My worst accident.

With Mr Whoppit. *(Nick Skinner)*

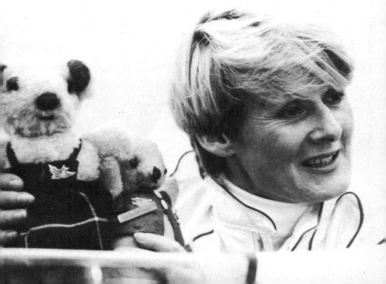

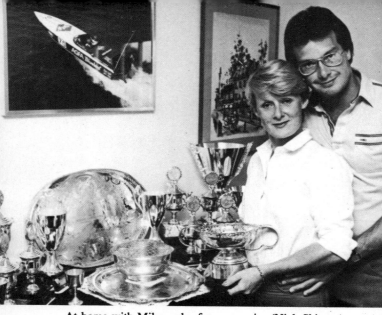

At home with Mike and a few souvenirs *(Nick Skinner)*

New Zealand 1, current champion in New Zealand and the boat I race out there.

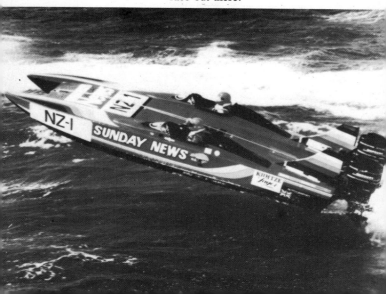

sure, but it was a good tale to tell when it was late in the evening and the ashes of the open fire around which we were sitting were glowing in the darkness.

Dad made a somewhat bizarre agreement to pay the Australian Ministry of the Interior £1 a year in rent for Lake Eyre for as long as he wanted to use it, which gave him exclusive rights. Elsewhere he had been hindered at times by other would-be record breakers. Even without his rental, I reckon he would have been safe from anyone but a fool or a saint in such a cruel, parched place as Lake Eyre.

He also arranged that the owner of the only sheep station in the area and his wife would prepare some of the meals for the team and give us access to such facilities as they had. The sheep station was at Muloorina, and to reach it from Lake Eyre you just drove several miles across the scrub of the desert as there was no road anywhere near. They had the only running water available to us. It was pumped from a nearby creek and contained a brown sediment which you had to wipe off your body whenever you had a shower. Clothes came out of the wash tinted with a soil-like pigment. The owner was called Elliot Price, a man then in his mid-sixties, I imagine, thick-set, bronzed and tough as they come. He was what an Englishman thinks an Aussie should be. Originally he had worked in mining but he saved his money and eventually put it into sheep farming. I was told more than once that he was illiterate, and equally often I heard that he was a millionaire. Both proved to be correct. While we were there he advertised blocks of Donald Campbell salt, cut from Lake Eyre, in one of the national papers. He was selling them at £1 each and was overwhelmed with orders, so that he made a few thousand extra bucks out of our presence. In fairness, I must also say that he was a first class sheep farmer. He had pens for thousands of sheep, mechanised shearing sheds and equipment to sort and bale the wool.

One day I thought the caravan in which I lived had

exploded. Outside, I found that what I had heard was the blast of a shotgun. One of the men had shot a six-foot deadly brown snake which was just slithering under the caravan. Right from the start I had never got into bed without first lifting the sheets to make sure that no lizards or cockroaches had taken up residence before me, but from then on I was doubly careful. And I never put my shoes or slippers on without shaking them out first. I was sweeping the floor one day and could not understand why the dust and litter was moving without the brush touching it. It turned out that I had swept up a scorpion from somewhere inside the vehicle in which I slept.

During the time we were at Lake Eyre and in Adelaide, quite a family spirit developed between the fifteen of us who made up the party. At the end of an exhausting and often frustrating day we would often eat at Mr and Mrs Price's home. It was rough and ready, but it's amazing how the most ordinary food becomes a delicacy when you are living and working outdoors all the time. There was an evening when everyone was heartily tucking into a lamb casserole and one of us commented, 'Nice bit of lamb, Mr Price.' 'Glad ya' like it,' he said. 'I found this one dead in the creek. I reckon she'd been there a week but she looked all right when we'd brushed off the maggots.' There was a sudden clank of pommie knives and forks as we all decided that the lamb was not quite such a treat after all.

Not only did the team have to eat but the men needed clean clothes every day, so Tonia and I were turned into glorified housemaids. We washed and ironed their shirts, darned their underwear and socks and made their beds. On our not infrequent retreats to Adelaide we had the same routine and, in addition, the catering to think about. It was a basic introduction to housekeeping for which I have always been thankful and, as a bonus, it meant that Tonia and I were working in partnership so that I was able to get much closer to her than previously.

156

Until then I had felt that she was Father's wife rather than my stepmother. I may be doing them an injustice but I felt that their relationship was so important to them that I fitted in only where convenient or necessary.

Tonia enjoyed being Mrs Donald Campbell and all that went with it and for a length of time she played the role very well, giving Dad all the support she could. Her theatrical background made her a ready subject for the photographers as she stood alongside Father, and she always had the quotable quote for the press on the big occasions. While they were married she did not do nearly so much cabaret work as she had done before, but this was not a sacrifice she made on Dad's account as much as a choice: she wanted to be part of the record breaking set-up. If the truth were told, I do not think Tonia would do anything unless she wanted to.

Sunday was always a day off for everyone but there was no form of recreation at Lake Eyre. Quite often some of the men would go kangaroo shooting with the Australian soldiers who were helping us with the track. I hated the idea and found that I developed an antipathy towards the men who spent their spare time in this way. On one of these hunts they shot a female with a baby in her pouch and brought the baby back to the sheep station. We had no idea how old it was, but even then it was three feet tall and its tail was as hard as a rock. The poor little creature was obviously lonely and so latched on to a PR girl who was there. It hopped around after her wherever she went and really became her pet.

On another weekend there was a barbecue in Marree, the local town about eighty miles away. A gang of us went in one of the Land Rovers, provided by the Rover Car Company back in England. With no roads to follow it was a rough ride, though it did give me a chance to see some more of the sunbaked heart of South Australia. It was all very sad. The place had an atmosphere of death about it. Everywhere there were bones of animals which had died in the drought conditions, whitened in the sun. There were skeletons of last year's victims of some beast of prey, slowly falling apart. There were carcasses – half-eaten, half decayed – and vultures were hovering waiting for us to pass so that they could return to continue gorging themselves. The death of any animal always hurts me and I know that I shall be told, as I was told then, that it's all part of nature. For me that is neither comfort nor excuse. My humanity demands that I feel pain at any unnecessary death and if what I saw in the desert is just to be accepted as part of nature, then nature itself is contaminated with the greed and violence which causes so much suffering in the world.

By the time we reached Marree I needed the music and dancing of the barbecue to raise my spirits. For £1 you drank as much as you liked and ate as much as you could – though I suspect the meat was aging kangaroo, judging by its toughness, and the team concentrated on the liquor. It takes a lot to frighten me but I don't mind admitting that I was scared out of my wits on the journey back to Muloorina. We were strangers, it was dark by then and all the men were as pissed as parrots. I had no idea how much alcohol they had managed to put down. We careered across the desert, bumped over dried-up water courses, went through one or two streams which somehow were still flowing, and even crashed through a dingo fence at one point. Despite its insect and reptile guests, the caravan seemed a safe haven after that journey.

As it rained at Lake Eyre once in a lifetime and there had been a heavy fall immediately after Daddy announced his intention of attempting the world record there, we could reasonably assume that we were safe from any further rainfall. Father's dreadful luck again turned against him. After the initial storm there had been several more in the time between his decision and our arrival, which was almost two years. In advance of our coming the army had prepared an excellent nine-mile course. Scarcely had the team settled in than further rain fell.

Weather changes very quickly in less temperate climates and we had not had time to get organised on the lake when the wind began to rise and someone spotted the twisting upcurrent of dust which shows the approach of a cyclone. We had two aircraft there; one belonged to Dad and he had chartered the other to carry equipment. He was anxious to get both out of harm's way and shouted to Ken Burville, the pilot in our party, to take the Apache and that he would take the Aztec. I was confused by the approaching storm and the haste with which everything was happening. 'Come on, you come with me,' he called, and the two of us ran to the plane, just grabbing what we could of our more important possessions and equipment on the way.

Breathless, and relieved to be in the plane, Dad began the take-off routine at once. Flaps, steering, lights, wheels – all the points on a pilot's checklist he went through in double quick time. No runway was needed as we could taxi across the hard salt, even though it was bumpy in places. In next to no time we were off and could look down behind us at the advancing storm. At about a thousand feet, without any warning, the door on my side of the plane flew open. It was as though someone was outside with a giant-size vacuum cleaner. The noise was incredible and everything that was not attached was sucked out and gone: cushions, maps, pens, a cardigan of mine, Dad's sunglasses, the odd bits of this and that we had grabbed as we rushed to the take-off – all gone in a second. I had my belt on but I was being pulled by an invisible force towards the wide open door. My hair was being tugged and was uncontrollably sticking out towards the door and it felt as though a powerful suction pump was pulling the flesh of my cheek in the same direction.

Had Dad not seen the danger and clasped his arm

around me very tightly I'm sure I should have gone. We completed our short hop – and thank goodness it was no longer – with the door swinging open and closed. Dad had an arm around me and flew the plane at the same time. When we touched down at Muloorina he told me that we had dropped 500 feet in altitude while he was wrestling to keep me on board and control the plane which was seemingly in a spin. It put me off flying for years, and can you wonder!

Next day, when the cyclone had passed, the soldiers set to once more and prepared an alternative course which they had ready within three weeks and then, on the evening before a record attempt seemed likely, the heavens opened once more. This time it was much more serious as Bluebird and all our technical stores were in tents well out on the lake. By the time Father and Leo reached Bluebird she was already in six inches of water. There was no choice about it, they had to get her back on higher ground. Dad had had little enough chance to drive Bluebird on the salt in favourable conditions; now he had to cope over a flooded salt surface which was becoming softer in the darkness and a gale-force wind. Bluebird, of course, had no lights so a Land Rover on each side escorted her and ahead there were other Land Rovers at intervals with their lights on to guide the convoy to the causeway. It was a delicate operation and it took more than three hours to get her safely above the level of the lake. The rainstorm was so heavy that it put an end to any lingering hope of tackling the record in 1963.

My journey home was as different as anything could be from the outward one. I was with Leo and Maurie who treated me with far more gentlemanly courtesies than a tomboy like me deserved. My father had given me some money to spend, which was rather unusual, and during a stopover in Fiji I bought my first transistor radio. Being an engineer by nature, Leo wanted to know exactly what each knob did, and why, before he would

160

advise me which one to buy. He went through every radio in the shop to make sure that I got the best. All the time I was feeling sorry for the shopkeeper dealing with two English tourists wanting to spend six dollars while there were twenty other customers with far more expensive purchases in hand and cash at the ready.

Those of us who had been in Australia knew that the team had readily accepted months of unremitting hard work in appalling conditions of heat and discomfort, that my father's dedication and courage had always been beyond question, and that where more money was needed it had been forthcoming. The fact remained that we had nothing to show for all the effort, and what the newspapers and the public wanted was a record. Several major sponsors shared this loss of confidence in Father and Bluebird and others wanted to take over the running of the project as a condition of continuing their support, which Dad, of course, was not prepared to accept, and so they too withdrew.

Dad's disappointment and annoyance were obvious in his expression and manner in those last days before most of us came back to Britain. I am not sure whether to call it determination or cussedness which motivated him to continue. Whichever it was, he set off on a quest for an alternative course. In the end he had to admit that Australia had nothing better to offer him than Lake Eyre, and all he could hope for was fewer misfortunes when next he went there.

I did not go on the 1964 expedition but know that it was even more spartan than the previous one had been. The party was smaller and for much of the time lived in army conditions and on army rations, as much of the backing from industry had ceased. Although Bluebird had been carefully washed down after each run in 1963 and before the storage period in Adelaide, when Leo saw her again there was rust in her bodywork and corrosion in her electrics. He and Maurie had an uphill task and when it was done and they reached Lake Eyre, the rigours of the surroundings had in no way lessened. The blazing sun, the energy-sapping heat and, perhaps most of all, the constant plague of flies made survival an achievement quite apart from attempting the World Land Speed Record.

The mishaps and misfortunes which followed were almost like a re-run of the first visit; twice the trailer taking Bluebird out onto the lake broke through the surface, wheel imbalance presented Dad with some terrifying moments, there was a fault in the throttle linkage and in this place where they said rain came once in a lifetime there was rain again. More than once courses which had taken weeks to prepare were made totally useless in downpours lasting only minutes.

Leo Villa in his book *The Record Breakers* says that the second visit to Lake Eyre was the only occasion in all his years of challenging for world records that he remembers any ill-feeling within the team. There were whispers that Daddy had lost his nerve and, when he had to have treatment for his persistent back trouble, his physical fitness to drive was questioned. It was an unhappy phase but, I think now, explained more by the physical and mental stress under which they were all living, than any real inadequacy of the people involved.

With more than a little of the do-or-die spirit about it, Dad decided he had waited long enough and was going for a record on 17 July. It was a Friday – a day on which he would not normally run – Bluebird was at her best, the weather was ideal and, though the surface was not as firm as he would have liked, it was better than it might be if he delayed. Tonia gave him a kiss, wished him well and handed Mr Woppit – now kitted out in Bluebird overalls and with a St Christopher medal – to Dad. The record attempt was on.

On the outward run the surface conditions made great demands on Dad's strength and skill, but his speed was high enough to put the record within his grasp. As the team at the turn-round carried out their duties they felt that he was tense and grim and unusually silent. Leo was concerned that when the turn-round was complete Dad was sitting in the cockpit gazing into the distance as though he had no part in what was going on. Afterwards he described how while this was going on he had a vision of my grandfather, who assured him that all would be well. What he said brings out both the mystique of the bond between my father and Malcolm, and also the fear he felt as he faced a hazardous second leg.

'OK, Skipper, we're ready when you are.' Leo's words brought Dad back to reality. As he roared away he knew he was driving on a track which no man should have dared to use. Bluebird was balanced on the razor's edge of disaster. As he approached the measured mile the thing he most dreaded happened – the surface collapsed. The wet salt acted like a giant brake and he had to overrun the engine to 110 per cent of rated power to sustain the challenge. The car vibrated frantically as rubber was stripped from her tyres. Only confidence in his machine, in his crew and in himself, and the indomitable spirit he had inherited from Grandfather, drove him on. The end was success – or eternity. From all accounts my father suffered the immediate sense of anti-climax which all record breakers know. He had done 403.1 mph and become the first man to travel on four wheels at over 400. He could not believe it.

What had been forgotten by most people in all the aggravation at Lake Eyre was that Father had set his heart on breaking both the land and water speed records in one calendar year. The enthusiasm of the Australian people about the new record rekindled that ambition, which had never been far from Dad's mind. As the convoy made its way back to Adelaide the streets of every community were lined with cheering people and in Adelaide itself there was a triumphal procession in which he drove Bluebird to a reception in the Town Hall. Later that year, back in London, she took part in the Lord Mayor's Show.

Five months of 1964 remained for Father to notch up a unique double. Leo and Maurie had to get the *Bluebird* jet boat ready for the attempt, while Dad had to decide where it should be made. Considering that she was by then ten years old and had been subject to enormous stresses in record breaking and being transported around the world, *Bluebird* proved to be in surprisingly good shape. Finding a location was less easy. The people of Barmera, on Lake Bonney, 150 miles from Adelaide, were willing to provide a boathouse, slipway and accommodation if the record attempt took place there. The team moved in but the lake was not really as long as it needed to be and, once again, the weather turned out to be unpredictable. Dad did his best as the whole community had been so hospitable but, with the days of 1964 running out, on 8 December he decided that he would have to find another lake.

The urgency of the quest was matched by the eagerness of the town of Dumbleyung, in Western Australia, to play host to the event. Lake Dumbleyung would not have been Daddy's first choice but when he had seen it, and the willingness of the community to assist, he gave orders that the whole *Bluebird* entourage should be taken by train the 1,600 miles from Adelaide to the new site. Leo described the place as a 'wild and scattered township in the centre of the vast barley and wheat-growing area'. It is about 140 miles southeast of Perth.

Imagining that any world land or water speed record could be established without difficulties would be to cry for the moon but Dumbleyung had a problem which Father had not come across anywhere else – ducks. The lake was thronged with them and the team had to get special permission to shoot some before the attempt on the record could be made. Apparently, it turned out that one shot before each run was all that was necessary as this sent clouds of them on their way, and almost all of them lived to tell the tale.

With nine days of the year to go Dad had his first run on the lake but conditions were poor and they continued to be for several days. On Christmas Day Tonia, Daddy and a friend of his called Lloyd Buley flew to Perth for a break but left instructions that the whole team should go to the Dumbleyung Hotel at 1.30 p.m. Unknown to them Dad had laid on a splendid Christmas dinner, and a couple of hours later Father Christmas arrived. With a seasonal 'Ho! Ho!' and shouts of 'Merry Christmas' all round, he produced the largest sack you could imagine and a beautifully wrapped present for everyone. It was Dad. For him something like that would have been almost as important as getting a new record.

The days between Christmas and the end of the year were littered with disappointments. Whenever there was the slightest chance of a run everyone would be alerted, usually to be stood down an hour or so later. The wind, known locally as the Albany Doctor, would sweep across and whip up six-foot waves on the lake in next to no time, and one attempt was frustrated by the failure of the timekeeper's equipment.

December 31 looked miserable from every point of view and in despair Tonia and Dad left again for Perth. Within minutes a water skier came ashore to tell Leo that the centre of the lake was as calm as it ever would be. A message rushed to the airport brought them back and within half an hour they were all set to go.

Leo knew how much depended on the next few minutes and recalls how he hesitated before giving the word to go. He had lived through the struggles and disappointments, he had shared the heartbreak when water or weather conditions had robbed them

165

of victory just when it seemed theirs, and he knew how many lives had been lost in this business because of a fractional error of judgement. When he knew the time was right, and disregarding the impatience of those around him, he gave Dad the all clear. With the two runs complete he had a new record of 276.3 mph and with three hours of daylight left in 1964 he became the only man ever to win both records in one year. I do not think anyone will ever achieve that again.

10

Father was now public property. His backers were quite naturally cashing in on their association with his success, Australians were proud of the honour he had brought to their country, in Britain he had joined the line of national heroes to which Grandfather belonged, to the rest of the world his attainments were the ones by which others were to be judged. The consequence of such popularity is that people feel they possess you. They think that what they know of you in public is the whole of what you are. In private, people such as my father have as many contradictions, failings and idiosyncrasies within them as the rest of us. Sometimes the newspapers, radio and television of his day made Dad out to be a swash-buckling tearaway who did not give a damn for anything or anyone, or, at other times, they portrayed him as a pale imitation of Grandfather who had lost the nerve to see through his record breaking plans. The people who worked with him knew him best. To them he was a very professional and scientific driver; someone who needed courage and incomparable persistence to overcome the mishaps and disappointments which beset him on the way to his goals. To me, he was a strong, kind man who had the sort of personality which could transform any group of which he was part. He was not just the fast-living Romeo.

Between his marriages Dad certainly had plenty of girlfriends. He was never secretive about them, though. He would bring them home rather than have clandestine meetings in London, and quite often I would tell him what I thought of them. More often than not, because he was supposedly part of the rich and famous set, women would seek him out as there was a certain kind of kudos in being escorted or entertained by Donald Campbell; and, being a very normal man, if what he needed was offered him on a plate, he could not say no. He was at a stag party in a nightclub when he first saw Tonia, but it was she who followed up the contact with a phone call the next day. He loved fast cars and flying light aircraft, and was always game for a trip to the continent or wherever.

Certainly the break-up of his marriages – to Daphne and then to Dorothy – was not because of an association with other women. The truth is that he was obsessed with record breaking so was away from home a great deal, and when he was there he was surrounded by racing people and all the talk was of boats and cars. Daphne and Dorothy both wanted something more out of a marriage than that, and both knew that they had qualities to bring to the relationship of which my father seemed scarcely to be aware. But then, what man possessed by such a compulsion would ever be easy to live with? It would have been totally out of character if he had arrived home each evening at six-thirty, put on his slippers and sat down to watch television. I do not think either my mother or Dorothy would have wanted that, but there was a middle course which, sadly, Father missed with both of them.

By the end, Dad's marriage to Tonia was deteriorating, and for the last few months they were living apart, though keeping in contact. Like Daphne and Dorothy, Tonia had to adapt to playing a supporting role to Bluebird and speed. She wanted more of the limelight for herself than either of the others, though, and would never really have come to terms with being away from her role as an entertainer. It could be that these qualities led Dad to hope that he could succeed with Tonia where he had failed before, and maybe that is why the rift with her seems to have been more painful. I saw a little of their ups and downs: I would hear raised voices, and one or the other would not be around for a day or two, and then quietly reappear as though nothing had happened.

Though his relationships were very liberal, towards me he was rather Victorian. He was very formal, and again and again quoted that saying, which I think most children of that day hated, 'Little girls should be seen and not heard.' He took it very literally, too. I was expected to eat my evening meal with them and any guests they were entertaining, but I was forbidden to initiate any conversation and allowed to speak only when someone spoke to me. He seemed to delight in having me around, though, and always wanted me to welcome anyone who was visiting us at the door, take their coats, see they had a pre-dinner drink, and make sure they signed our visitors' book. But I loved him because he could be such great fun. Sometimes when we had a party of friends in for a meal, he would come into the dining room with a bowler hat on, a chiffon scarf around his neck, a cigar in his mouth, an umbrella in his hand, and football shorts over his trousers. He loved dressing up and would have people in stitches of laughter. I shared in the enjoyment, but I always felt it was done for them and not me.

Because I was never sure whether he was going to be the disciplinarian or the clown, I was terrified of him. He was so strong and able that he literally seemed like God to me. I never remember sitting on his knee to be cuddled, as I saw other children do with their fathers.

Though he could be good company socially, there was an insular quality about him in his professional life. Unlike Grandfather, Dad was not competitive. Malcom used to race at Brooklands in the blood and guts days when drivers were killed almost every Sunday afternoon. With Dad it was him and his machine against the clock. Dad was a much softer, gentler character, and

169

by nature a loner. I have more of Grandfather than Dad about me in both looks and temperament. I need to win even if it's only at Scrabble or Trivial Pursuit!

I was too young to have any real idea how my father's non-competitive nature affected his business life. I suspect that he could have made a great deal more money than he did, but we always lived in a pleasant house with staff to help run it, I had food to eat, clothes to wear and went to good schools, so I was luckier than many children. Our standard of living changed from one year to the next, though. When Father was doing well there was plenty of everything, and we could go anywhere, but there were times when we seemed to be more careful, and my guess is that these were when income had fallen or expenses on record breaking had shot up.

Although we lived comfortably and Daddy was a public figure, there was no snobbery about him. He believed that the dustman was as good as a Duke. At Christmas, you would find him in the kitchen with the postman or one of the gardeners enjoying a Bluebird Cocktail. This consisted of vodka and Blue Curacao, and was his own invention. Some people said that he was pompous, and I know what they meant. He had a clear, well-modulated voice which had a note of authority, his appearance was smart and he had an air of command, but these things were part of his nature and the product of his background rather than the product of assumed self-importance. He had a great sense of the value of other human beings regardless of their status, and an equal dislike of slovenliness or a lack of ambition, whether it was in a pauper or an aristoctrat.

My father was a great admirer of Winston Churchill and delighted to smoke a cigar in public to promote his Churchill image. He was a showman, and when he took part in the television programme *What's My Line* not only would he smoke a cigar but he also wore a monocle. We would be watching at home and killing ourselves with laughter, because we knew his eyesight was as good as anyone else's, and that it was all part of an image he wanted to put across.

His television appearance which I remember best was when one evening I was quite definitely told to sit down and watch TV – which was unusual. Mr and Mrs Botting, who worked for us at Abbots, were with me as Dad and Dorothy were out, and they said I would be interested in the programme which was about to begin. It was *This Is Your Life* – the seventh edition ever transmitted by the BBC – and Dad was the subject. He had gone with Dorothy to the theatre where she was appearing and, as she came on stage, Eamonn Andrews also walked on with the red book and captured Dad for the programme. I was very proud and still have the book which the BBC gave him that January evening in 1956, but I feel slightly sad that I was not there to be part of it.

If appearing on *This Is Your Life* gave Dad pleasure it was no greater than the pleasure he found in giving people presents. Mostly they had to be surprises – like the car which he gave Leo after he set his first record – and always they were generous. After a lean spell, when money began to come in his first thought would be to go to Reigate or London and come home with presents for everyone in the house. One Christmas, being a tomboy, I had made it clear that I wanted a bow and arrow. When he returned from his shopping trip I identified my present and most of the others, but there were two which meant nothing to me, and had no labels on them. 'Who are these for, Dad?' I asked. 'Ah, that one,' he said, 'that's from Donald for Campbell.' 'And what about the other one, then?' I persisted. With a chuckle he replied, 'That's from Campbell for Donald.' The strange thing is that when I was at boarding school and other girls received parcels from home, there was never one for me. It was as though he enjoyed giving big flamboyant things but forgot that a few sweets in the post would be important to a little girl.

171

He also had firm ideas about the way you addressed people. He liked me to call him 'Father' or 'Daddy' but not 'Dad', though I have to confess that it is as Dad I generally refer to him now. Quite often he would call me 'Georgina' and would add, 'That's what you were christened.' As I grew up, if I had a boyfriend who rang me and said, 'Oh, good evening. Can I speak to Gina?' in imperious tones he would say, 'She is Georgina, if you would not mind referring to my daughter by her proper name.' The poor fellow would hang up and run a mile! I used to cringe with embarrassment. He had an old-fashioned sense of propriety which he would not let go of.

Looking back, I cannot understand why I did not rebel against all this. I was not in any way a well-behaved child but, for some reason, accepted quite philosophically Father's style of doing things. Very often I feel that in the present day world young people are the poorer for not having these niceties of etiquette instilled in them.

Daddy, like Grandfather, was very concerned about how Britain was run and what her standing was in the world, and, had he lived, might well have gone into politics, I think. His friend, Edward Du Cann, stood for the Conservatives at Barrow-in-Furness in an election in 1955 and Daddy supported him at some of his meetings. Sir Edward, as he now is, says that Dad spoke 'simply, directly and movingly'.

In the election the next year when Sir Edward won the Taunton seat he says Daddy spoke for him in the village hall at Wrantage, just outside the town. He was taken there in a Jaguar driven by the chairman of the local Conservative party, Mr Bageot Kite, who had been well known in the west of England as a rally driver. Daddy caused roars of laughter when he began by saying, 'Ladies and gentlemen, you may be here to see the holder of the World Land Speed Record and the World Water Speed Record, but this evening I have been terrified by being driven at the speed at which your chairman tackles country lanes!'

Edward Du Cann and his brother Richard had both taken part in the *This Is Your Life* programme about Daddy. Sir Edward, a stranger to the area, had been selected as prospective candidate for Taunton a few days before the programme, and his picture had been in the local papers. He reckons that being on *This Is Your Life* strengthened his position in a by-election which took place a month later.

Side by side with his public concerns it always strikes me as being inconsistent that someone as practical and rumbustious as my father should have been interested in spiritualism. Towards the end of his life he would go to see mediums, thinking that he could make contact with Grandfather. Yet he was not a religious man in any other sense, and never went to church. His interest in spiritualism had begun soon after he married Daphne. One cold morning they invited the milkman in for a cup of tea. The morning's newspaper was lying on the table with a headline on it concerning some spiritualist event. Dad remarked that it was all a lot of ridiculous nonsense, to which the milkman replied rather quietly, 'Then you must know all about it.' Dad felt a complete idiot. All he knew was what he had read in papers and magazines.

The milkman turned out to be an experienced medium and the conversation led to him inviting Dad and Daphne to his house for one of his sittings. His only condition was that they should come with open minds and not in a spirit of hostility. Until then, both my mother and father had thought of spiritualism as a group of old ladies sitting round a table, holding hands in the dark. Peter White, the milkman, who was to become quite a close friend, showed them something quite different. He would go into a trance whether the surroundings were in darkness or daylight, his face would become rather ethereal and he would say the most wonderful things which were

173

inspiring and comforting. It was all from the teaching of the New Testament, Dad recalled.

Peter had accompanied Daddy and Daphne when they made their sales trip to Belgium soon after the war, and being with him for several weeks had provided the opportunity for them to see more of his spiritualistic qualities than would otherwise have been likely. When they were sharing what Dad described as the 'ferocious' hospitality of the crew of a British merchant ship in Ostend, Peter drank much more than he should have done. In his drunken state they were amazed to hear him carrying on a fluent conversation in French with a member of the crew who came from the Channel Islands – and they knew that normally he could not speak French.

Later on, while the three of them were sightseeing in Bruges, my father became particularly interested in a collection of armour and ancient weapons in one of the museums. The place was thick with atmosphere, and Mother gradually became aware that Peter had an unusual expression on his face and the hair on the back of his neck was standing out horizontally. She realised that he was going into a trance and quietly led him outside, leaving Daddy totally preoccupied with the exhibits.

A similar thing cropped up on the way home from that trip. They had just passed the North Foreland and, though it was a beautiful sunny afternoon, the sea was very choppy. Dad was at the wheel, Mother was holding tightly to a ladder to avoid being thrown about and Peter was securing himself by pressing himself against the side of the cabin. Without warning and quite naturally he slipped into a trance. He sat down on a highly polished seat with his legs crossed under himself and his arms folded across his chest looking rather like a Buddhist monk. While they were hanging on for grim death Peter was perched on this polished seat looking as though he was glued to it.

I am a realist, and spiritualism has no appeal for me,

but if it provides some sort of strength or solace to other people, I would not want to question or ridicule their belief.

Within Father's make-up there was also a superstitious quality, and while very different, spiritualism and superstition may well go hand in hand. At times his superstitions were annoying. He would not have anything green in the house nor was anyone allowed to wear green clothing, which could limit the ladies' wardrobes quite considerably. At one stage he insisted that Leo should get rid of a green felt cap he was wearing and replace it with a blue woollen one. He was paranoid about thirteen people in a room and should there by accident be thirteen people for dinner, he would call the butler to come and sit down with us. He would also be most devious in preventing a third cigarette being lit from a single match.

Another thing which sometimes annoyed people about him was his phobia about being wished good luck. He regarded it as an adverse omen, and would say *'merde'*, which is, I believe, a vulgar French way of repudiating good luck and means shit.

Like many sportsmen he had certain items of clothing which he felt went along with success. He had a pair of shoes which he always wore for record attempts, and he had developed a ritual which he went through before he got into either his Bluebird boat or car. Dad had inherited many of his superstitions from Grandfather. Malcolm would never do a record attempt on the 13th, and avoided Fridays. Indeed, the whole Bluebird legend is based on a fairytale about happiness and superstition. All of us have carried a small silver plate with an enamelled bluebird on our cars and boats. When my father was at Lake Eyre and Lake Dumbleyung, in Australia, he wore a blue leather race-suit, and had a navy blue blazer with bluebird buttons, and wore specially tailored blue shirts to sustain the myth that blue is associated with good fortune.

I do not pretend to understand Father's or Grandfather's superstitions. I believe that you make your own luck. It is careful planning and a bit of shrewd manoeuvring which pays dividends at the end of the day. When I started racing I took Mr Woppit because he was a mascot which Dad had used, but now he has become more precious as a token of Dad's courage and achievements. He is such a prized possession that now I leave him to watch from the tow-truck. Originally, Dad also had a partner for him, Mrs Whacho, and a wooden carving of the Polynesian god of happiness, Mr Tiki, whom he also took on his record runs.

Whether Mr Woppit went ski-ing with my father I do not know, but certainly he skied a lot during the years that he was married to Tonia. He had introduced her to the slopes on their honeymoon. Until then she had little interest in sport. Two months later he rented a chalet at Courcheval, in the French Alps, and took virtually the whole team. No one could understand why I did not want to go. In retrospect, I think it was in part a protest against Father's new marriage. I had nothing against Tonia, I just wanted to be me. Much more, I preferred to stay at home and mess about with ponies, which were becoming more and more important to me. But just think of it – being angry because I had to go on a ski-ing holiday! It proved to be a memorable holiday, and ski-ing is now one of my greatest pleasures. My most outstanding memory of that first Alpine holiday is of a fondue party which Father organised on top of one of the mountains late one night. Of course he invited the man who owned the ski-lift along, and his daughter, and inevitably they opened the ski-lift for us to get up, and later we all came down carrying torches. It was romantic and exciting.

In those days, even more than now, a winter sports holiday was something special, but I could be just as happy doing ordinary things. Our butler and his wife had their own television room, and I used to sneak off and have an hour or two watching programmes with them. I say 'sneak off' as Father did not allow me to mix with the staff. He used to say that 'familiarity breeds contempt' and I had no idea what he meant. Occasionally, I would spend some time with some of them, unknown to him. This happened most frequently when his marriage to Tonia was breaking up. We lived in a large house and, having neither brothers nor sisters, I was lonely.

The people who really helped me through my periods of loneliness – and there were several of them – were Leo Villa and his wife, Joan. I think Leo always felt that I had a rough deal and he went out of his way to allow me to share in the happiness of their home. Maxie and I stayed there quite often when Dad was away, and their son Tim was the nearest thing I ever had to a brother. I was there on Leo's birthday one year – he was sixty-three, I think – and when I found out how old he was, I just said, 'Nobody gets to be that old.' They never let me forget it. I think it says a lot for Leo and Joan that although they included me in so many of their family activities, they did so in such a way that I do not think Tim was ever jealous. They were wonderful people.

Joan worked in a shop in Reigate which sold sports goods and Leo used to go into Reigate from Abbots to have lunch with her. If I was at home, I would sometimes go with him and I always had fish and chips. He had a Sunbeam Talbot with a running board along the side, and when we got back to Abbots he would let me drive and stand on the running board himself to make sure that my erratic steering did not lead us into trouble. Those lunchtime outings with Leo and Joan were so simple, but they stand out among the happiest recollections that I have of my childhood. All my life Leo contributed to my happiness. I knew him for longer than I have known anyone else: he was there from my earliest days, and when he died in 1979 I knew I had lost my most precious friend.

My schooldays were a background to all these events. I went to various schools, and I do not look back on any of them as being happy places. Typical of my reaction to school was one morning while I was at De Notta School, in Reigate, when Gillian McKenzie and I decided that we had had enough. As the rest of the school went into assembly we slipped out of the front gate. We walked and walked for what seemed to be miles. We must have been so obvious to anyone as girls playing truant with our polka-dot dresses, boaters and blazers. We had got as far as the top of Reigate Hill – which was not very far, really – when we saw the Games Mistress coming up in her car and she called to us. Until that moment I don't think it had occurred to us that we would be missed, still less that a search would begin. As soon as she shouted we realised that our freedom was threatened, and we ran for our lives. We got back into Reigate before she cornered us, and we had to be taken back to school in her car in disgrace.

However irksome school may have been, the compensations at home continued. Soon after Daddy and Tonia got married, they bought a house which Dad had always wanted called Roundwood. It was quite close to High Trees, the school at which I lived for a while after my mother and father separated. It was a much larger house than Abbots, with a big garden, and surrounded by a copse: hence the name Roundwood. It was a lovely house but did not have a happy atmosphere, and I never really felt that it was home. When term finished just before our first Christmas there in 1959, and I arrived home, Dad told me I was not to go to the top of the garden. I did not dare ask why, nor did I dare to go there. On Christmas Eve he took me to the forbidden part, where a stable had been built. Inside was my Christmas present – a pony. It was just like heaven to me. I was so excited. I'm not sure which I thought was more wonderful – Dad, or the pony.

For the rest of the day I don't think I left my pony.

She was all that I could ever have wanted. I went to bed eager for it to be morning so that I could go up to the stable again. I must have been in this excited half-sleep when, in the early hours of what was Christmas Day, I heard Dad in the garden shouting. It took me a few seconds to appreciate what was going on. My pony had got out of the stable and Dad was trying to catch her. From my window I could see in the moonlight that she was going like the clappers – through the flowers and the fish pond, across the lawns and the tennis court. Father, breathless and exhausted, was chasing her all the way, with a head collar in his hands. He would not have known which end to put it on! I quickly put some clothes on and ran out into the garden to help, as I felt responsible for what was happening. 'No, no, I can manage,' Father said, motioning me away, 'Bloody things,' he went on, 'dangerous at both ends and bloody uncomfortable in the middle.' Father had no interest in riding, and that was the last time I remember him having anything to do with the pony.

When next I changed schools Daddy arranged in advance with the headmistress that I could take my pony, and that he would pay an additional fee for her to have a stable during the winter months. Never had I returned to school more willingly than when we set off from Roundwood, the Land Rover loaded with my baggage as well as all the equipment I needed to look after my pony, which was in the horse-box behind us. The school was at Tring, in Hertfordshire, and I can remember going round Marble Arch, in the centre of London, and up the Edgware Road with the pony whinnying all the way.

It was winter but, when we arrived, the headmistress said that my pony would have to be outside in a field. I told her that Dad had made special arrangements, but she would not budge. I went to a phone box and got through to Father who very soon got in touch with the headmistress. They fell out over the phone and Father gave me instructions to pack all my belongings and leave the school at once. It was all very dramatic, but Father felt that the headmistress had broken her word, and that he was not prepared to tolerate it. The only snag was, I was in the front line. Poor Tonia was left with the task of finding an alternative school for me, and finding it within a week. That was how I came to be at The Warren, near Worthing.

With so many changes at school I never settled down to my studies as I ought to have done. The only subject which I really enjoyed was geography because I always wanted to travel, but even in that I did not manage to get an 'O' level. I found it hard to concentrate as I preferred riding, rounders, tennis, swimming, netball and, most of all, lacrosse. Lacrosse, I think, is the most physical game ever invented. Fancy arming kids with a stick with a net on the end to play a game with virtually no rules. You go for the throat, beat your opponent to death and then trample all over her! What I missed in formal learning at school I think I have made up for in the breadth of experience which I have had, and I think I can hold my own in conversation with almost anyone I meet in adult life.

Another problem at school was that most of the other girls seemed reluctant to make friends with me. I could not understand this at the time, but I think it may have been because I was the daughter of someone well known. They assumed that we were richer than their families or would not want to do ordinary things, or they were perhaps jealous of the advantages they thought I had. Little did they know! Being the offspring of someone who is famous is not easy, as both father and I found out. The only time things became a bit easier was when Dad broke a record and telephoned school asking that we should have a special half-day holiday to celebrate it, but my popularity was short-lived.

One school friend whom I remember is Carol Bass, but not for a very creditable reason, I'm afraid. Both of us

180

had ponies at the school we were attending at Worthing, and they were kept at the commercial stable next to the school. We were about fourteen and allowed to ride without supervision. Neither of us enjoyed school, and one winter afternoon we decided that it would be much more fun to ride over to her parents' summer cottage at Wittering than go into lessons. Without anyone noticing, we went through the wicket gate between the school and the stables, saddled our ponies, and set off.

It was further to Wittering than we had realised, and before long it became dark and started to rain. We rode in single file along the road, and were constantly dazzled by the lights of oncoming cars. It is amazing how quickly you lose your bearings in such conditions, and quite soon we had no idea how to get back to the school and even less idea how to get to Wittering. We were wet, cold and hungry but we did not give in until quite late in the evening, when we saw the lights of a large house some way from the road. It was ridiculous really, as all the time we assumed that we were being very grown-up and no one at the school would have missed us. We rode down the long drive to what turned out to be a stately home called Parham Park.

We rang the doorbell and, when the butler came, asked if we could use the telephone. We explained that we had been riding and were lost, and wanted to hire a horse-box to take us and our ponies home to Wittering. With that dignity and detached efficiency which you will only find in the traditional English butler he accepted our story, invited us in and showed us where the telephone was. In truth he must have been agog at the sight of two drenched kids turning up on the doorstep at ten o'clock at night. We were talking about hiring a horse-box but we did not have a penny between us.

None of our calls produced the help we wanted, and while we were on the phone the butler went away and made us a cup of tea. He brought it in the finest bone-china cups, and I know I disgraced myself by pouring

181

mine into the saucer and taking it outside to my pony. The owner of the house was out for the evening so, while we were drinking our tea, this very kind butler made one or two calls to people whom he knew owned cattle lorries, but was no more successful than we had been.

Suddenly his old face brightened, 'I've got the answer,' he said. 'I'll ring the police – they'll know who can help in this emergency.' We listened as he recounted our story to them. 'They're coming over themselves right away,' he said, putting the phone down, 'Our police here are very good, you know.' Carol and I were shattered. The truth had dawned on us simultaneously. They were not coming for the ponies, they were coming for us. We had been reported missing by the school.

Before long there were lights in the drive, and two patrol cars with blue lights on their roofs pulled up outside the front door. Facing the police was bad enough, but now we knew we also had to face the wrath which awaited us back at school. To make things worse, at that moment the owner of the house arrived home and was quite concerned when he saw police cars outside. The explanation which his butler gave sounded like the plot of a children's adventure film, in which Carol and I were cast as villains.

Our host could not have been too displeased as he offered to keep our ponies in his stables overnight, and while we waited for someone from the school to come and collect us he showed us a little more of the house. It was very big and there was one room which was full of braces of pheasant which had been shot on the estate, and there were lots of guns and deerskins, I remember.

Back at school, we gathered afterwards, there had been total panic among the staff when they realised we were missing. Over the evening meal the head had increased the anxiety by suggesting that we might have had a mishap on the Downs, been kidnapped, or killed in an accident. After such hysteria, when the truth came

182

out it was inevitable that our punishment should be pretty severe, and the clever way it was handled ensured that we were regarded by the other girls as outcasts who had 'let the side down'. All very jolly hockey sticks! For weeks we were not allowed to ride, were denied all other privileges, and were humiliated by having to take classes and our meals with the seven-year-olds in the junior school.

Dad's reaction to the incident was most interesting. He was very angry and gave me a good dressing down when next I saw him, but all the time I felt he was doing what was expected of him rather than what he sincerely felt was necessary. He knew that we had put ourselves at risk and was concerned that we should understand this, but deep down I think our initiative and daring appealed to him. Maybe I wasn't a son but I do have some devilment about me!

When all this happened I did not know my mother, and she and Father had only the slightest contact with each other, but she has told me in more recent years that she found Daddy's attitude to my education very annoying. When I was at home she feels he was too strict with me, but at school he seemed to think that as I was a Campbell I was above the rules, and the powers that be ought to fit in with me. In the end it was my mother who made sure that I took a secretarial course in Hampstead and, though I did not enjoy it, it has been useful in the years since.

I was not the instigator of all my adventures. At one stage my father owned a very smart motor cruiser called *Golden Seal*. Dad, his spiritualist friend Peter White and I were moored in what I suppose is the most prestigious spot in sailing anywhere in England – right outside the Royal Southern Yacht Club, on the Hamble river, between Southampton and Portsmouth. The tide runs very fast there, and to manoeuvre a boat demands a lot of skill and care. *Golden Seal* had dual controls – one set on the bridge outside, and the other in the warm and dry. Somehow the controls on the upper deck jammed and Dad could not change to neutral or reverse. Within minutes we were bearing down on a much smaller boat whose occupants were screaming and shouting with fear. Father was leaping from one control position to the other, and Peter and I were out on deck with fenders, boat hooks and lines trying to avoid a collision. Through sheer physical strength we managed not to run down the other craft, and with sighs of relief sailed away from a scene of near disaster.

Such an incident never disconcerted Father for long. He soon suggested that we sail across Southampton Water and into the Beaulieu river, to visit his old friend Lord Montagu. The short journey took longer than we expected as we managed to run onto one or two sandbanks on the way, and getting free took time. The weather was not very good, and as it was getting on in the evening, we decided to moor for the night and pay our call on Edward Montagu in the morning.

Between us we prepared a meal and then the men started a game of cards and the booze came out. I went to my cabin, got into bed and before long was sound asleep. During the night a most awful crash woke me and, as I came to, I realised I had been thrown out of my bunk onto the floor. I tried to stand up but couldn't as the boat was lying on her side. The same thing had happened to Dad and Peter, but it had not hit them quite so hard because the brandy and port had numbed their senses. There was an increasing smell of gas and we found that the Calor gas container had fallen over and was leaking. Father at once assumed the role of skipper again, and in his best Uppingham accent ordered us to abandon ship. That was easier said than done. What had happened was that the tide had gone out while we had been asleep, *Golden Seal* had grounded and then toppled over, and abandoning her involved jumping into mud to our thighs.

To complete the farce Edward Montagu was just rowing across what water remained to come and rescue us. Never has the sight of a peer been more welcome! The story that Donald Campbell, the world's most respected boating man, had been found with his motor cruiser lying on her side in the mud because he had forgotten the tide never got into the papers, and I think it was just as well.

Throughout these years I had never met my mother and when I did it happened by accident. I was about sixteen, I suppose, and Daddy and Tonia took me along to a cocktail party to celebrate the opening of a new stud farm close to where we lived. Not only was I glad to go because I loved horses so much, but it was the first cocktail party to which I had been. It was very crowded, and whenever I was in public with Dad I always felt people were staring at me. 'My dear,' he used to say, 'the time to worry is when they don't.' That particular day I tugged his sleeve and said, 'Daddy, they're doing it again – they're staring at me, and there's one lady over in the corner and I wish she wouldn't. She just keeps looking and looking at me.' Dad looked across the room and then back at me, and after a pause said, 'That lady is your mother.'

I had learned by then to take anything in my stride. I was surprised, of course, but certainly not embarrassed or annoyed. Had I been embarrassed, or stopped to think for a moment how she or Dad, or Tonia for that matter, might feel, I would not have said with blind innocence, 'Shall we go and say hello?' The three of us greeted her and her husband and spent most of the rest of the evening with them. I could not understand why their conversation was so stilted. It only occurred to me years later that when Dad and I accepted our host's invitation to have a swim in his pool we had put my mother and Tonia in a difficult position. Dad's willingness to go for a swim at that moment was perhaps slightly mischievous.

I had first been aware of my mother's existence when I was at boarding school at about eight or nine years old. Dad was at that time married to Dorothy, who had meant so much to me, and as far as I was concerned was my mother. At school, however, in that painfully direct way which children have with each other, another girl said, 'You've got two mummies, haven't you.' 'No,' I said, 'I've got a mother and a grandmother. Of course I haven't got two mummies, stupid. You can only have one mother.' When next I was at home I told Dorothy about this remark, and very sweetly she sat on my bed with me and explained that she was not my real mother, but I had a real mummy who was no longer with Daddy. We had a hug and a kiss and the only time it bothered me was when I received two birthday or Christmas cards both saying 'With love from Mummy'.

Having met my natural mother we kept in touch. As she had racehorses and a stud farm we had a shared interest which helped us to get to know each other. I shall always be disappointed that she was not more closely involved in my childhood, but I love her and feel no animosity towards her. She is now married to a charming man, and they are blissfully happy. I always enjoy going to visit them, but I do hope that one day we can be brave enough to talk about those missing years. Mother's main fault is that nowadays she is too caring about my racing and my love life!

Daddy knew that my only ambition was to be with horses. The obvious thing was to be a groom. One of Dad's special friends was Pat Smythe, who was Britain's top showjumper then, and I had aspirations in that direction too. It was natural then that when I left school he sent me to be trained to teach other people to ride. The course was at Lewes, in Sussex, and at the end of it I qualified as a British Horse Society Assistant Instructress. The course was well worth while. In the early stages we had classroom instruction on horse and stable management in the mornings, riding all afternoon, and then private study in the evening, so we had no time to spare. Once the staff knew you had an aptitude for the job you were promoted – if it is a promotion – to mucking out, grooming and exercising the horses, and later on still, training them to jump. To learn to teach people to ride the instructor would have twenty-four horses for the class of twenty-five, and each of us would have to take a turn at teaching the rest of the group. I remember standing in the centre of the circle saying, 'Trot, please', or, 'Fiona, keep your toes in,' or, 'Bottom down, please, Amanda.'

There was something odd, which was perhaps good for me, in moving from the limelight into which I had been thrust because of who my father was, to doing hard and dirty work in a stable on cold winter mornings. Behind the façade of success and fame there are always the simple basic things which we all have in common.

11

If anyone had told me beforehand that one day I would slap Tonia's face, I would not have believed them. She was the woman to whom Daddy was married, and therefore my stepmother, and I accepted her. We had some happy times together but there came an explosive moment when we argued and I hit her. It's not something of which I am proud, but I think she used it to achieve something which would otherwise have been impossible.

The row blew up one weekend when I was at home while I was working in the charter department of British Eagle Airlines. This was my first job after secretarial college, and during the week I shared a flat in London with two other girls. My father had given me a car and I went home each weekend, and by the time I got home on Friday evenings I was feeling all in. How the argument began I have no idea, but it was about a bottle of shampoo, I remember. It was as trivial as that. I suppose I was going through a difficult period with a job that was making great demands on me, and a home which didn't feel quite like home any more. Anyway, voices were raised, tempers aroused, harsh things were said, and completely spontaneously I slapped her face.

She made no attempt to scold me or be reconciled, or to hit me back, but rushed upstairs to my father's study, screaming, 'Either she goes, or I go!' Minutes later, looking somewhat concerned and dejected, Father appeared and before he could say anything, I said, 'You don't have to make the decision – I've made it. I'm going.' My bravado did not leave him a chance. Within an hour I had packed my belongings and was away.

Already, I had arranged that when the summer holiday period arrived I would leave British Eagle and go to do reception and secretarial work for Norman Buckley, a long-standing friend of Father's and holder of various water speed records, who owned three hotels in the Lake District. After leaving home I brought my plan forward, gave up my job in London and went to work for Mr Buckley. I was mainly at the Low Wood Hotel in Windermere, but also at the Royal in Bowness. It was there that I met Helmut, a gorgeous, fair-haired, blue-eyed German who was their head waiter. I fell head over heels in love with him, and at the tender age of seventeen decided that he was to be the man of my life. So much in love were we that at the end of the English summer we both took jobs at the Park Hotel in Arosa, in Switzerland. I think the reason I gave Father for going to the Continent was that I wanted to learn to speak German, but this turned out to be impossible as almost all the time I was working with Italians.

My first job was in the laundry at the Park Hotel, where I used to press what seemed like an endless stream of gentlemen's shirts. Maybe that is why I am such a fussy shirt ironer now! Sweltering over an iron, all I could see ahead of me for hour after hour was a wall of newly laundered shirts, and whenever I asked if we could have a window open as I was near exhaustion, my highly-strung Italian colleagues would object. When the shirts were done, they had to be laid out on tissue paper, and the housekeeper used to say, 'You must take them up to the room yourself, then you'll get a tip.' It was ironical, as at home we had a butler and a maid who did all this for us, and there was I – for the love of Helmut – ironing shirts for a living.

The housekeeper at the hotel was a young French girl and, although she was my immediate boss, we got on quite well. One day she came down to me in the laundry with some urgency to say I was wanted on the telephone. I had been following in the English papers, which reached Arosa a day or two late, how Daddy had been getting on with his World Water Speed Record attempt on Coniston Water, and knew that things had not always been going his way. Knowing this, and knowing that no one would ring me from England between eight-thirty and nine o'clock in the morning unless it was very urgent, I think anxiety must have registered on my face at once. The housekeeper had no idea who my father was but when she saw my worried look, she said, 'I'll come with you.'

It was my mother's voice on the phone, and instinctively I knew what she had to tell me. She said that there had been an accident, but she would not say whether Dad had been killed or not. Whether she genuinely did not know, or whether she was sparing my feelings, I have no idea, but I think she knew. I did not need to be told the rest. I was choked, I was numb. I was cold. I had always known that this could happen, but now that it had I could not believe it. I could scarcely speak. My eyes seemed to be fixed in one immovable staring position, but my tears just would not come.

No one had clean shirts that day, and there were no clean sheets either, as the housekeeper dropped all her chores, took me by the arm and looked after me for the rest of the day. Together we went out in the snow as I wanted to wear some lovely boots which Daddy had bought me in Courcheval the previous winter. I had always wanted them: they had hair on the outside and looked as though you had a couple of Shetland ponies wrapped around your feet. I gazed at shop window displays of expensive watches and fine jewellery, but saw none of them; the mountains were clear as crystal but seemed to be shrouded in mist – for my wonderful father was dead. I was alone.

During the afternoon I heard on French radio that he

had been killed, though the confirmation was unnecessary. The more painful thing was standing in the departure lounge at Geneva Airport the following morning waiting for my flight home, and seeing all the newspapers on the stand with the headline 'Campbell est Mort'. People were talking about the accident and about my father. To them it was a news story, an event which happened yesterday. To me it was a bereavement. Poor Helmut was with me, and I felt sorry for him. We had thought we were so much in love, but he knew so little of me and nothing of the bonds which bound me to Daddy. He had no experience which could have taught him what to say to someone in such depths of grief, any more than I would have done had our roles been reversed, but in a kind, quiet way he supported me. I stared in disbelief at those headlines, saying to myself again and again, 'Don't look. Don't torture yourself,' but I was transfixed by the horror of it all.

As I was not at Coniston during those fateful days at the end of 1966 and over New Year 1967, I am dependent on what other people have told me and what has been written for my impressions of what went on. Certainly the two years between achieving the double in Australia and his final attempt on the World Water Speed Record at Coniston were ones of uncertainty and frustration. Popular interest no longer saw the ultimate in human achievement as speed on land or water, but as the exploration of space and landing a man on the moon. Even so, the American Art Arfons and Craig Breedlove had pushed the Land Speed Record up to 600 mph using rocket and jet cars, but my father still felt it as something akin to a duty, as an Englishman, to be the fastest man on both land and water. He had Ken Norris begin design work on a rocket car which would be capable of breaking the sound barrier at sea level, and enlisted the support of the Jamaican Government in staging the event. Despite all his efforts his backers were not interested and the scheme had to be dropped. He also thought for a time

191

of a new record for the mile from a standing start, but Dunlop felt that the high cost of producing the tyres needed for such a venture could not be justified.

It was in this moody, restless frame of mind that Dad and Tonia moved from Roundwood – the house which he had wanted for so long before he bought it – to Prior's Ford, in Leatherhead. Just before they left Roundwood Dad put the Bluebird car, the *Bluebird* jet boat, and the model of the projected rocket car on display in a marquee on the lawn. It was as though he was saying to the friends, industrial contacts and the press whom he invited, 'This is what I have done, now give me your interest and support to do still more for Britain.'

His spirits plunged still further when a rally driver called Peter Bolton took his place driving Bluebird on a demonstration run at Debden Airfield, in Essex, and accidentally hit the accelerator. The car careered through a hedge, across a road and went broadside into a field of corn. Peter Bolton was not hurt but repairs to Bluebird were estimated at £50,000 – and all because Daddy was poorly on the day of the Debden Gala.

Even though he was less than his buoyant self at that stage Father's inventiveness knew no bounds. He set about putting a reasonably priced, family-size jet boat on the market. He called it the Bluebird Jet Star. It was the kind of invention which could have made him a millionaire several times over and solved his financial problems, but again the effort was doomed to failure.

Suddenly, almost without warning, he decided to have another go at the World Water Speed Record on Coniston Water. *Bluebird* had seemed to have finished its record breaking days after Lake Dumbleyung, but he took her out of retirement for the attempt. Leo was doubtful about the idea, though Ken Norris was more optimistic. The Beryl engine was replaced by a smaller but more powerful Orpheus, and to ensure that a spare was available Dad bought a complete Gnat fighter just to get the engine. Other parts, too, turned out to be useful, and the fuel pumps, starter and some of the controls as well as the tail were used in the updated *Bluebird*.

The modification went better than anyone could have foreseen and by November *Bluebird* and the team were at Coniston. From that point onwards, though, the enterprise seems to have turned sour. Their workshop consisted of nothing more than a tarpaulin stretched over some metal poles, and it was both wet and cold. Connie Robinson had by this time moved from the Black Bull to the Sun Hotel. Her care proved to be essential to everyone's morale. Bluebird's air intakes appeared to be sucking in water which caused her to flame out, the engine suffered from fuel starvation, she seemed to be too low in the water at the bows and so on. It was all very disappointing and time-consuming. There was some media interest, though in the deteriorating winter weather there were mumblings of discontent from some members of the press corps about the delays, and this did not help.

As Christmas approached, still no serious attempt on the record had been made, and a day or two before the festival the Swiss timekeepers announced that they were going home for the celebrations. On Dad's insistence the team too dispersed to their families, leaving him alone at Coniston.

True to his nature, Dad made a couple of trial runs while all the specialists were away, depending only on local support. When Leo returned he was very displeased by this and took Dad to task for the unnecessary risks he had taken with no qualified rescue team in attendance. 'So what?' he replied. 'It's doubtful if the rescue boat could get to me in time if anything did happen.'

It was 4 January 1967 before conditions were good enough for a record attempt and everyone was assembled at dawn. Leo recorded in his book that he said to Father, 'Doesn't look bad at all today, Skipper.' In a strangely detached way Dad replied, 'You'd better get everybody out to their stations,' but he seemed to have no inclination for a chat or a joke as he usually did before an attempt on a record.

At 8.42 a.m. *Bluebird*'s engine was started. The record attempt was on. Leo says that when Daddy passed him he was going very fast indeed and *Bluebird* was rock steady. Soon, in the distance, he saw the plume of spray which showed that Dad had put on the water brake. Normally he would have spoken to Leo on the radio to check that his wake had died down and that the surface was ready for his second run, but this time all he seemed to want to know was his speed. It was 297 mph and, to Leo's consternation, he said over the radio, 'Stand by. I'm making my return run.' A moment later he said, 'Full power,' and he was roaring northwards across the lake. There were some slight ripples but all seemed to be going according to plan. Then, when *Bluebird* was well into the measured mile, Dad's voice was heard saying, 'She's tramping . . . the water's not good . . . I can't see much . . . I'm going . . . I'm on my back . . . I'm gone'. And then silence.

It was to this silence that I returned. I know that the feeling was not mine alone, and I am not exaggerating when I say that there was an atmosphere of national sadness. I felt unworthy to be the daughter of a man who had occupied such a place in the hearts of so many people in Britain. In a way the public reaction to the accident was comforting, yet no one could get inside me and know exactly what it meant to me, and perhaps I did not know myself until some years afterwards.

My mother and her husband met Helmut and me at Heathrow and very thoughtfully they had arranged special customs and immigration clearance for us so that we were not besieged by reporters. The four or five days we stayed with them at their home at Capel, near Dorking, were dreadful. Each news bulletin and every newspaper had something about Dad's accident in it, yet there was nothing new to be said. Divers went down and unsuccessfully searched the lake for his body, and there was talk of recovering *Bluebird*. In my distress, I was quite illogical. I knew that no one could survive the kind of accident he had, but I was hoping against hope for a miracle. For me, and I expect for other people who have to cope with personal tragedy, such irrational thinking is a kind of buffer which the mind erects between feelings and reality. I heard little of what went on at Coniston at this stage. One thing I do know is that Leo was in bed suffering from shock for several days after the accident.

Tonia had been in London when Dad was killed and after a couple of days I decided to go to see her. It was an awkward meeting. We had not been in contact since I left home and I knew that she and my father had been far from happy over the previous few months; both had tended to go their separate ways and pursue their own interests and relationships. I went to her flat in Dolphin Square and found her very much the grieving widow, stretched on a sofa, heavily sedated, and surrounded by people being very sympathetic, few of whom I knew. I was doing my duty but I felt superfluous. I cannot recall what conversation we had; probably very little for there was nothing to be said. Quite soon I left, knowing that the meeting had done nothing to help either of us.

Even more painful than my call on Tonia was a visit which I had to make to Dad's solicitor, Victor Mishcon. He telephoned me at Mother's a day or so after the accident to say that he needed to see me as there were complications about the will. Apparently, Grandfather had left £20,000 in trust for me with Father as the custodian. He was able to use the interest but the capital sum was to come to me when Father died. At some stage Father had managed to get the capital released and made use of it in his business and record breaking. He obviously intended to repay it but his unexpected death meant that he did not have the opportunity to do so. Mr Mishcon explained that I could make a claim against Dad's estate to recover what was mine, or I could sign a document relinquishing all rights to it.

I was only seventeen, in a complete state of shock and without anyone to advise me. I could not comprehend what was going on. Having given me this information, being my father's solicitor and executor he could give me no further guidance and certainly could not act for me. I did not make a hasty decision, but, later on, surrendered any rights which I might have had under the trust which Grandfather set up. My only reason for this was that I did not want to appear to be suing Dad. His memory was far too precious.

As Daddy's body was never found there was no funeral. None of us would choose to go to a funeral, yet I feel that in coming to terms with the greatest tragedy I could ever know I lacked that moment when I could say, 'Goodbye and thank you', and 'I hope I'll live up to the traditions which you set'. In a way, I suppose, a funeral is therapeutic. Although we know that our nearest and dearest have to die sometime we are never ready when it happens and the less so when it is unexpected. Going to a funeral lets uninhibited grief and the comfort of happy memories react on each other to salve the hurt.

Some while later there was a memorial service at St Martin-in-the-Fields, but it was public and formal and I had to be on my best behaviour. Tonia told me before I went that I was not to cry. I felt total disbelief in the occasion. The family sat on one side of the church and the public on the other, rather like the guests of bride and groom on separate sides at a wedding. Tonia chose to sit with the racing team rather than the family as, she said, Daddy had called her 'Fred' and regarded her as part of the team because she helped when he was attempting a record. Afterwards we went back to Tonia's flat where we ate sandwiches and sipped coffee, rather as though we were at a party.

Dorothy, my first stepmother, had returned to New

196

Zealand after her marriage to Dad broke up, and remarried. She was pregnant and confined to bed with a very bad cold when Dad was killed. She remembers press photographers pushing their way into her home wanting to take pictures of her, as though she was of some interest after all the years that had elapsed. We had not seen each other since she left Dad, but she says her thoughts were for me that day. She remembered, too, that while she was married to him, she went to see an old fortune teller in Ireland and Daddy wanted to know what she had said about their marriage. Dorothy teased him and would not say, so he changed the question and asked whether she had said that one day he would have the good luck to be blown up in his boat. He had hated seeing Grandfather die painfully and slowly and, in a sense, envied John Cobb's sudden death. If he had to go, Dorothy thought, then this was the way he would have wanted it to be.

My mother heard the news of the accident on the radio. Within herself, she refused to believe it. But then, there was only one Donald Campbell and only one man attempting to break the World Water Speed Record on Coniston Water. The previous evening they had spoken on the phone, as they occasionally did, and he had said, 'I'm hoping to have a go tomorrow . . . Look after that little 'un of ours.' He knew that the higher the speed the greater the risk, but, for me, it was a reassuring thing that my welfare was uppermost in his mind.

One of the most moving tributes to Daddy was the one at Courcheval. Late in the evening on the day of his crash many of the ski instructors and villagers who had known him went up the mountain and formed up in the letters DC. In the darkness they lit torches and stood in silent tribute to a man who had found so much pleasure in their area. It was as though his name was engraved on the slopes on which he had skied, and the gesture reflected the mark which he had made on so many people in so many places. At first he had simply been known as Sir Malcolm Campbell's son, but as his attainments began to match those of my illustrious grandfather he was acclaimed in his own right. Mistakenly, particularly in Australia and New Zealand, he is often still referred to as Sir Donald Campbell. A knighthood was never his, though he was awarded the Queen's Commendation for Gallantry within a month of his death. The Australian Government have honoured him with a memorial at Lake Dumbleyung and I have to confess that when I unveiled it, just as I was about to pull the curtains back the thought crossed my mind that it would be dreadful if they had engraved *Sir* Donald Campbell on the stone. To my relief, they had not.

For me it is hard to assess my father as someone who pushed back the frontiers of human experience in science, engineering and sportsmanship by driving fast cars and boats, because to me he matters in personal terms so much more. Two minutes before the accident he was saying how dangerous what he was doing would be, yet he did it, and that is true courage. Yet throughout his career he was absolutely clinical about safety. There were risks enough without taking chances, he felt, and he was meticulous about every precaution which could be taken. The tragic thing about him is that his finest hour was his demise.

A great deal of publicity was given at the time to a story that while playing cards on the evening before the accident Dad had turned up the ace of spades and then the queen of spades and interpreted it as an omen of death in the family. Whether he did or not is a matter for conjecture, but if it did happen, I cannot think that it would have in any way influenced his attitude to the record attempt.

In recent years there have also been suggestions in radio and television features that he did not wait for clearance for the second leg of his final attempt on the record because he wanted to end his life. It is true that he was emotionally unsettled and that he had financial difficulties, but to make such a suggestion shows a greater love of sensationalism than of truth, and indicates that the people concerned never knew my father. For him, every problem was a challenge, and around every corner the Bluebird was waiting. Few men or women have had more optimism or a greater love of life than Daddy.

When it became clear a few days after the crash that all hope was gone, my mother suggested that I go back to Switzerland. I think she found it difficult having me and Helmut around, and I understand her feelings. Goodness me, if I suddenly had a seventeen-year-old daughter whom I had never really known inflicted on me, I think I too would want to ease her back into her own way of life as soon as possible.

Back in Switzerland I did not have the heart to return to my job. I found bed and breakfast accommodation in Arosa with a lady who was very good to me. She was motherly, though always treated me in a very businesslike way as a paying guest. Day in and day out I went ski-ing, remembering that it was Dad who had first introduced me to this incomparable sport, and that in his last letter to me he had asked me to reserve some dates later in the month so that we could all go to Courcheval again after he had set his new record. Helmut had returned to his job at the hotel but gradually we drifted apart and made our own lives.

When I returned to England, some weeks later, I divided my time between my mother's and Tonia's homes but my mind was numb and I cannot remember people saying things to me or doing things for me. The accident had robbed me of my father whom I loved, the home which one day I could have returned to, and the financial security I ought to have been able to depend on. In a vague way I started looking

199

for a job, having decided that I wanted to work with horses. It was eighteen months before the final papers by which I relinquished my right to anything from Grandfather's trust were completed, and by then I was married.

12

The Bluebird of happiness never seemed further from my grasp than in the months following Daddy's death. From the earliest days that I can recall I have been keen on ponies and horses, and at that stage my interest in them became a form of escape. I thought about going back to work at British Eagle Airlines but I think having to stand in a queue for a ticket on the tube and being jostled in London crowds would have been too much for me. I was emotionally very unsettled, and the slightest thing would make me cry. Quite harmless remarks which people made would bring tears to my eyes if they were said in the wrong tone, if I dropped or broke something I would burst into tears, or if I was uncertain of where to go or what to say crying was my immediate response. It was a very difficult time for me, and I felt that working with horses would give me a chance to care for something other than myself, and the response which you get from animals would in part fill the void I was feeling.

My British Horse Society training course at Lewes had given me some qualifications to offer when I applied for jobs. The first one I considered was in Canada. I saw the advertisement in *The Times*. It was asking for a girl groom to work with a Master of Foxhounds, and live in with the family. It also offered a free flight across the Atlantic. After writing a letter and sending my CV to the agency I was offered the job, but the snag was they expected me to sign a contract saying I would stay for two years. If I did not do so, then I would have to pay my own fare home. It was a longer commitment than I felt I could take on, so I asked if they had any alternative openings.

Their suggestion was that I should contact a Mr and Mrs Muirhead, who lived in Hampshire, and who were in need of a girl groom to live with them as part of the family. When I went to see them I was impressed straight away. They lived up a two-mile private road in the middle of nowhere. The nearest village was Droxford, which is in the lovely Meon Valley between Alton and Fareham. Mr Muirhead was an ex-cavalry officer in his mid-seventies, and his wife was some years younger.

Although I had relinquished any claim on the trust which Grandfather had set up for me, I inherited £500 from Daddy and with this I bought my first car. It was a Triumph Spitfire, and I got endless pleasure out of it. Somehow it seemed to give me individuality and dignity as I drove through the country lanes around Droxford on my days off.

The Muirheads had the most amazing selection of dogs in and around their home, from mongrels and strays to pedigree ones which would not have been disgraced at Crufts. Mrs Muirhead knew how much I needed warmth and a quiet style of life so, to my surprise, suggested that I should get a dog of my own. 'Could I keep it here?' I asked incredulously. 'One more isn't going to make any difference,' was her cheery reply.

Even before Mrs Muirhead made her suggestion I had made my mind up that when I had a dog she would be a Labrador bitch. I did not like the way dogs sit there and lick themselves all the time and catch hold of your leg, and so forth. The local saddler's shop in Droxford had a small-ads board and on my next half-day I went to see whether anyone was selling the kind of dog I wanted. I was unlucky, but the owner of the shop put me in touch with a kennel at Sonning, near Reading, where they bred Labradors. It was, I suppose, the longest trip I had done in my sports car at that stage, but it was well worth while when I saw Lisa. She was quite small for a Labrador and a little bit nervous. She was just over a year old, but had been caught 'on the hop', as they say, in her first season, and had a litter of puppies. Fortunately, they were old enough to be left and within minutes I was handing over my money and Lisa was on a lead and chain on her way home with me. She jumped into the car and sat in the passenger seat looking out of the front as though she had been doing it all her life.

When you have a new possession, particularly when you are young, the first thing you want to do is show it to someone else. I called on Brian Hulme – Buddy, as I knew him – who had been a special constable with Dad at one time and had been married to my Aunty Jean, to show him and his new wife my lovely Labrador. 'I can't leave her in the car,' I explained, 'I must bring her in.' I had forgotten that dogs have a certain smell about them when they have been in kennels and took her into their very smart lounge. As you would have expected they admired her and said all the silly doggy things which we say, and then Buddy said, 'Coo, Gina, that dog doesn't half hum!' As gracefully as I could I withdrew, but Lisa and I had already become inseparable.

Like most Labradors, Lisa was playful and mischievous. Just as you were going to put your hand on her collar she would jump away, so I kept her tethered on a very long lead – 200 yards or so – in the garden or yard at Mr and Mrs Muirhead's which saved time if you wanted to catch her when you were in a hurry. There was also what I will call the sherbet incident. I used to like lemon sherbets and was foolish enough to leave several packets in the glove compartment of the car. Lisa sniffed them out and scattered the lot over the beautiful blue interior. I was so cross with her that day, and she knew it.

I had joined Mr and Mrs Muirhead in September 1967, and as the start of the new hunting season approached they thought their hunters which had been out to grass during the summer should get into trim for the opening meet. A local showjumper, Clifford Percy, had a full set of jumps and we arranged that he would give the horses a workout over his course once or twice before hunting began. Each time I rode one of the horses, and enjoyed the chance to do some jumping. Clifford Percy turned out to be a very gentle, easy-going man, with a great love of animals. That November he invited me to go to a bonfire party with him, and other dates followed.

When I first came to Droxford for my interview with Mr and Mrs Muirhead I had noticed what turned out to be the Percys' house. It was a lovely place with stables beside it which looked like the National Stud. To be honest, I was rather disappointed that the job I had come about was not there. Mr Percy senior was a very ordinary man who had worked hard and done well. Prior to the war he had sold milk from a pony and trap, but then when the war was over he got into the garage and secondhand car business in Portsmouth. He was a real wheeler-dealer. His money was in the business but he went there only to advise or abuse. Mrs Percy was a complete contrast. She was a quiet but strong country lady, who had a warmth and humility which I admired.

Clifford and I had a lot of interests in common, and most of all our love of horses. He already had quite a reputation as a junior in showjumping, and with his experience he gave me a lot of help and I began to enter local gymkhanas and horse shows. One of the things that impressed me about him at that early stage was how keen he was for me to do well, and I found that I was equally concerned that he should succeed. We got on extremely well, and in June 1968 we were married. I won't say that Lisa was my bridesmaid, but she sat at the back of the church throughout the service and came with us on our honeymoon. In the absence of Daddy, I was proud that Leo – Unc – was there to share the day.

Our first home was a flint cottage called Elm Farm, at Baybridge, not far from Droxford. It was almost uninhabitable when we bought it. It was damp and dirty, and the surroundings had been neglected. It had no hot water system or central heating, and outside there was a generator which provided electricity to a lead which was suspended around the wall on nails and coathooks and had a socket for a naked bulb here and there. The value from our point of view was that the cottage had fifty-five acres of land and a number of useful buildings with it, which we used to train horses. With lots of hard work and the assistance of the local builder we turned what was a rural slum into a pleasant and comfortable home.

The Percy family had built up a reputation for being able to break and train difficult horses which no one else could manage, and Clifford continued with this specialisation. Old Mr Percy, I was soon to discover, was a tidiness fanatic and would walk around with a pocketful of leaves and pieces of straw which he had picked up around the garden or the farm, and he preferred Clifford to be at home keeping things spick and span rather than competing in horse shows. I think my arrival provided the support which Clifford had always needed in showjumping.

With Clifford – or Cliffy as I used to call him – I probably had the most complete companionship I have ever had. We seldom argued and our horses were everything to us. We had eight very happy years together.

The best horse I ever had was Taurus. We saw him advertised in one of the horsey magazines for £250. He was a handsome five-year-old chestnut, and quite large. The owner was an old man: a schoolteacher who had bought him at an auction at Ascot less than a week before. He had a vet's certificate to say that he was sound in wind and limb but we were slightly unsure of him. We tried his jumping ability over a five-bar gate and were both stunned by the six feet of air that he left between himself and the top of the gate. At the price we were being asked, we decided he could be a real bargain.

Taurus proved to be somewhat sour-tempered at times. He would put his ears back and swish his tail sometimes when you looked at him, and half lift a hind leg as much as to say, keep away, but he had an engaging personality and I came to love him. Clifford's father was equally impressed when he saw Taurus tackle his small showjumping course. We turned him out into a field and, knowing how keen I was to get going with him, Cliffy said, 'Taurus is going to be for you. When he comes up from grass he's going to be totally your responsibility – you're going to school him, you're going to ride him, you're going to take him to his first shows.'

Our hopes for Taurus were to be dashed to the ground. When the time came for his training to begin he soon became lame and the vet diagnosed nevicular disease which is incurable. It means that the bone which the muscle rides over in the hoof becomes slightly degenerate and wears, leaving a rough surface for the tendon to ride over. Several years later, Taurus sadly died while under an anaesthetic. He was not insured and I had refused an offer of £15,000 for him not long before, because I loved him so much.

I cannot pretend that we made anything like a good living out of our horse business. To help out we kept pigs. They were not my favourite creatures and on the occasions that I had to feed them I was terrified. When I went into the field with a bag of the pellets which they ate, they would all charge at me and I was in danger of being knocked head over heels. The technique, I learned, was to move away from the herd as I began to scatter the food and hope that when I ran out they were grovelling on the ground with sufficient enthusiasm not to notice.

For all my dislike of feeding the pigs, nothing gave me more pleasure than seeing the piglets born. Among all farmyard animals pigs are the ones most despised but

I think this is mostly unjustified. As babies they are most attractive, and I even managed to make friends with the boar. In the end I could tickle his tummy and he would roll over like a dog, and I could sit on him and ride him round the field. He was wonderful, but unfortunately from the point of view of pig rearing as he became more and more friendly he became useless for the purpose for which we kept him. Having a pet boar running around the house was out of the question as they are strong and potentially very dangerous, so he had to go to the slaughterhouse.

Throughout our time at Elm Farm I never managed to reconcile the conflict within myself about killing animals for food. I know that a good farmer will always say you must accept the death of them along with the life of them, but I have never come to terms with this. I make no judgement about what anyone else does, but I am almost completely vegetarian in my diet. In any case, I think a vegetarian approach is more healthy than a menu overloaded with red meat.

As well as the boar, we had a sow who was rather a favourite with us. One of her litters had just been weaned and taken away from her, and on the same day an electrician came to do the wiring for a new stable block we had built. Cliffy and I went out late in the afternoon before he had finished. We were surprised when we came home at ten-thirty to find the electrician's van still there. As we got out of the car we could hear cries of 'Help' from the stable loft. Our pet sow was playing the deprived mother role and, thinking that the stranger had taken away her babies, was pushing, rubbing and oinking in anger at the foot of the ladder. He had decided not to face an irate pig and was stranded, and afterwards had the cheek to charge us overtime for the three or four hours he had been caught in the loft.

Though we never again had as promising a horse as Taurus we had some good second-rankers. Before I met Cliffy I had ridden at the White City, but our set-up gave me the chance to take part in shows all over the country. We always took several horses to any show and I would ride them in different classes depending on their particular strengths, and we had considerable success. Rosettes and trophies from the Royal Windsor Horse Show, the Bath and West, the Devon County and countless others accumulated in our dining room. I never really achieved anything in the Horse of the Year Show at Wembley but each time that I failed to win I resolved to do better next year. My favourite course was, I think, Hickstead which has an atmosphere all of its own, and Cliffy and I always felt that we were on home ground when we went there.

Representing Britain in showjumping abroad is as much a matter of your willingness to give your time and finance to the trip as a question of ability. At each opportunity we put ourselves forward and were able to keep the flag flying on various occasions in France, Belgium and Holland. My main disappointment about this aspect of my life is that I did not manage to reach Olympic standard.

Showjumping satisfied the need which I have to compete, but I have to admit that I used to get into very bad moods when the horses did not do as well as I knew they could. I think it was this unpredictability of the beasts which led to my gradual loss of interest. You could work and work to get one ready for an event and then you would open the horsebox at the venue and he could be lame, or coughing, or have colic, or something. I did not know how my future was going to work out at the time, but it seems that I eventually swapped the oats for the carburettor. And there's not as much difference in the cost as you might think.

Seen from outside, I suppose Cliffy and I had an ideal marriage. We lived, ate, slept, worked, drank together, and shared so many interests. I was not keen on having children so the fact that the most personal side of our life broke down was not a serious problem, but I began to feel that if I was not prepared to move I would be mucking out horses forever. Cliffy was quite happy with this prospect, and I do not blame him for that. I was the one who was restless and wanted a new and wider challenge.

It was Tonia, who had moved to the United States to develop her career as a cabaret artist after Dad's death, who quite unwittingly provided the way out for me. During the summer of 1978 she phoned to say that she had a cabaret engagement for a month in Portugal and asked whether I would like to go with her. Our relationship had been decidedly frigid, but maybe she had sensed that while the peace and quiet of a rural life in Hampshire provided the healing which I needed immediately after the accident, I had become bored. I had not had a holiday for years and the thought of exchanging the smell of horse dung and the mushrooms growing under my fingernails for a few weeks lying in the sun was irresistible.

By this time Clifford and I had sold Elm Farm, at a very good price, and were living in a flat. When I returned I told him how I felt, and he was devastated. It is true that we had a good life together during the years which we shared but I needed more. He pleaded that we should continue as we were, but that would not have been good for either of us. Eventually he told me that he had been having quite a close relationship with one of the girls at the stable of which I had not been aware, so the dissatisfaction with our marriage was as much felt on his side as mine. He moved out of the flat, and we parted fairly amicably.

Looking back I can see that the move from my first marriage to the second was rather hasty. I think that this may have been because I had already met Philip Villa, who became my second husband, when I was still in my teens, though we had had no contact during the intervening years. He was Leo Villa's nephew and served his apprenticeship as an engineer with Leo and Dad. I used to chat with him in the workshop sometimes, but there was nothing more to it than that as he was already in his twenties and an age difference of five or six years at that stage in life means that you do not see each other in romantic terms. It was not until I was separated from Clifford and the divorce was going through that we met again. Both of us happened to go to the hospital at the same time to visit Leo in what turned out to be his final illness in 1979. The age barrier did not seem to matter any more, and an attraction between us, which had been non-existent when first we met, suddenly developed. It seemed the most natural thing in the world to meet again and have dinner together. Six months later we were married. My divorce from Clifford came through in January, I went to live with Philip in March 1979, and we had a July wedding.

Philip lived in a very old cottage at Effingham, between Leatherhead and Guildford, which he had rebuilt into a beautiful house. He had a very good job as a design engineer in the petro-chemical industry, and went off to his office in London each day. He was involved in oil-rig design and gas exploration in the North Sea, which was then at its height. I had decided to give up competitive riding as I wanted to be less involved with horses, but I had kept two young ones for my own pleasure which I stabled at Ranmore Common, about five miles away. My daily routine was to take Philip to the station, go to Ranmore to muck out and exercise the horses, do any shopping and attend to my domestic jobs. It was an undemanding life of freedom which initially I appreciated.

What had attracted me to Philip, I think, was his endless flow of ideas. He was a great guy and full of the highest aspirations. In his spare time he devoted his skills to making models. One of these was based on his theories about the future improvement of my father's last *Bluebird*, and he had plans to achieve the ultimate in Water Speed Records himself. On the face of it, it might seem that with his engineering qualifications and interest in maintaining the *Bluebird* tradition my marriage to Philip was the fulfilment of destiny and would have had Daddy's approval. I have never felt this way. In fact, I question whether my father would have been happy at the thought of me marrying someone who was a relative of one of his employees. Dad had very clear lines of demarcation between the family and the staff.

At about this time – again cast as the daughter of a famous father – I was invited to open a new wind tunnel at Imperial College, in London, which was to be named after Dad. Philip and I attended together and he lost no opportunity in talking about the revolutionary design and his plans to set up the outright record for speed on water. Just as we hoped, the college offered to put the model to the test in the new wind tunnel.

Students at Imperial did a considerable amount of work on Philip's brain-child. A craft with such a pedigree – Campbell and Villa – had to be taken seriously. Philip's faith proved to be misplaced, and the results were unimpressive. In fact he was so disappointed with the report that he never even showed it to me. I could understand how disappointing it was for him, but the way in which he then abandoned the whole scheme and never even bothered to make the improvements they suggested was beyond me.

Having done so marvellously modernising his cottage in Effingham, we moved a short distance to East Horsley, having it in mind to redesign our new property. The work was not as straightforward as it looked and again Philip lost interest. Philip's failing seemed to be that he would stumble at the first hurdle. If things did not come to him straight away he would rush off and do something else. Much though I appreciated and enjoyed other aspects of our life together, this tendency to give in was something I could not accept. In my family a difficulty was no more than something to be overcome.

If Daddy and Grandfather had given up at such an early stage they would have achieved nothing and not have been remembered, and poor Philip suffered for this.

Increasingly I came to feel that my new life was less satisfying than my former one had been. I no longer took part in horse shows and I missed the stimulus of the business side of what Cliffy and I had done. I think Philip did his best. He was abroad for several months at a time in connection with his work, and he would ring me most days and come home for the odd weekend when he could. He seemed to think that as long as I had a house and garden, and my horses, I should be satisfied. I had become a queen in a castle, stuck away out in the country, with only a motorised lawnmower for pleasure. That mower became very important. It was one of those with a seat over the roller, and you spin it round bends as though you were driving in a Grand Prix. In the summer months, almost every day I would put my bikini on and fly around the acre of lawn, just to have fun. It must have been intensely annoying to the neighbours, and we had the shortest grass for miles around! Finding pleasure in cutting a lawn said something rather sad about the remainder of my life at that time.

Even when Philip was at home, life came to have little more colour about it. Dutifully, I would be sitting at the station ready to pick him up at 6.35 p.m. He would arrive with his newspaper under his arm, we would go home for our meal, watch television, and he would fall asleep. And next evening would be the same. I'm sorry, but I found it boring.

Throughout my time with Philip his friend Michael Standring had regularly come to the house to do odd jobs on our cars. When Philip's car needed fairly major surgery Michael came for a whole series of evenings and I would get a meal for the two of them, and then they would be busy right through into the early hours. It was therefore natural that, when Philip was abroad, if I had

212

a problem with the car I would ring Michael. I always offered to pay him as Philip had said that he needed the moonlighting, but he declined. I was rash enough to suggest, when he was coming straight from work to do a repair which would take a couple of hours, that I would have something ready for him to eat, and this became our pattern.

Michael was several years younger than me. He was a handsome and athletic man, but with an abrasive nature. Some months before his wife had left him. Far from giving in if things did not go right, Michael had the sort of ego which drove him on and on until he succeeded. We were each what the other needed, and an affair started. Before long, my husband's friend who came to mend the cars had a greater interest in the bedchamber, and the interest was returned with warmth.

Whatever feelings I may have – and there are plenty – I cannot deceive people, and I simply had to tell Philip at the first opportunity that Michael and I had become lovers. I did not find this as difficult as I expected – perhaps because our relationship had become so formal and unexciting. Philip's reaction took me by surprise. Without meaning to, I had broken his heart. He was taken completely unawares and was distraught. Until that moment I had never realised how much I meant to him, but what puzzled me then, and still does, is why – if he loved me so much – he chose to go and work so far away for such long periods. I know that I betrayed Philip, and I am not proud of it, but he did not put an awful lot into our relationship. It was a milk and water existence which left me as a bored housewife in a pearly castle.

There was no time to find out whether our marriage could be saved, or whether there was anything worth saving. With Philip still reeling from the shock, I moved out and set up home with Michael at Priors Ford, in Leatherhead, which had been Daddy's last home.

13

It is not easy to say how my period of unconscious mourning for Daddy came to an end, or, indeed, whether it ever completely has done. Without any bidding people will recount what they remember of him, or tell me of someone closely associated with his efforts whom they knew. They remember the day of the accident and how they heard about it, and, more to the point, what they felt. Many of those who are younger and who were not alive in his day can, after a moment's thought, tell you something about him. I am proud that so many people want to share a little bit of his glory. A man who challenged and held at bay forces of science and nature as often as he did and with such determination, and who in the end was their victim, is worth commemorating. The facts of his life have been embroidered with stories and anecdotes but nothing can detract from the statistics in the record books, his contribution to nautical and motor engineering, and what he did for British national pride. While I am overwhelmingly pleased by all this, to me he is much more. I am held captive by the memory of him. I feel that I owe him a debt. His dynamism is still restless within me.

Over the years I have often been introduced as Donald Campbell's daughter, without anyone explaining who Donald Campbell was. I have been amused as people have reacted with a blend of interest, sympathy and fascination, and, in an intrigued tone, have said, 'Oh, really!' Then they have often followed up with the thing which gets up my nose: 'Do *you* do anything?'

My new companion, Michael Standring, played a very significant part in helping to lift me out of my despair and begin to do things. He was the manager of the spare parts department at a local car showroom, and I found it an advantage that he did not observe the social conventions nor have money, which had played such a part in my marriages. He was not influenced by the atmosphere in which I had grown up. Like me, he loved speed and had successfully taken part in Mini Clubman racing. He was a full-blooded man who liked to enjoy himself and, knowing something of the Campbell story, he was initially, I think, flattered to be looking after cars for one of the family.

Having been swept together on a wave of romance and passion, the reality of everyday life was less easy. With Philip I had been a pampered housewife; with Mike I had to get a job to help keep us. I cannot pretend that I liked travelling round southeast England selling tablecloths and napkins to hotels but it saw us through an otherwise difficult time. I called at places to which I had been with my father and seen him welcomed as an honoured client by the proprietor or manager – the Dorchester Hotel included. As a sales representative I might have to sit in reception awaiting the convenience of the housekeeper, only to be sent away with a message from her saying that nothing was required.

Weekends were not much fun either as Michael was nearly always playing golf. I thought about getting another horse but decided that this would keep us apart rather than provide an interest which we could share. One day, I said to Michael right out of the blue, 'Shall we get a boat?' He liked the idea and a week later we owned a sixteen-and-a-half-foot ski-boat, and she was immediately christened *Bluebird*. We had to buy a manual to learn how to drive her, and I remembered how Dad had set off down the Thames for Belgium with the instruction book in hand! We were completely smitten by our new hobby and in every spare moment

215

we were on the water. For me it was success, for Michael it took his golf handicap up from single figures to the twenties.

We had bought the ski-boat solely for our own recreation and entertainment – and we really meant that – but within our first summer we paid visits to many race venues to watch, and listen – and learn. Perhaps we made ourselves a bit of a nuisance at times by trying to run alongside the boats which were racing, but it was all good experience. Tiny thought she was, our 85 hp *Bluebird* was introducing us to the social and sporting world in which both my father and grandfather had been masters.

During this period it would have been easy to exploit my family connection and equally simple to conceal it by using a married name. I tried to be just myself, and, almost without exception, Michael and I managed to appear as interested onlookers. My inward grieving over the years had created in me a reticence which meant it was not hard to be alone when other people were socialising, and Michael was very understanding. I was aware of an increasing urge to compete but I needed to sort out my aims and motives much more clearly before anyone had any idea I aspired to be the third Campbell.

We talked selectively to people who had the racing knowledge and the idealism which had driven my father and grandfather on and on, and I'm told that as people got to know who I was they felt I had a superior attitude and was distant. I am sorry if this was so, but it was not part of any deliberate policy. In fact, I recognise this phase only now that I reflect on it some years later. At all costs I had to avoid the gin and tonic bonhomie in which I might hear yet again, 'Donald Campbell's daughter . . . what do you do?' And, although my international showjumping career had been quite impressive and no one had known that I was a Campbell, all I had to show for my interest in speed on water was an insignificant ski-boat scarcely worthy of the name *Bluebird*.

My father's philosophy had always been that it was everyone for himself or herself in life. I, too, believe that things do not come to you, you have to go out and get them, and rather than give in to my own uncertainties I knew I had to face up to them and make things different. I knew other people whose lives had been shattered by tragedy and who were fighting back, but somehow we always feel that our own grief is unique. The most hopeful thing was that I began to feel that offshore racing might be my release.

One person to whom I talked more than most during this sorting out period was Peter Armstrong, who had won the national 3D power boat championship in 1983. These conversations brought to a head the process of decision which had been going on in my mind. I might never do as well as Daddy or Malcolm had done, but within my own limitations I was beginning to believe that I was as good as anyone else and I cherished the hope that I might just happen to be better. My mind made up, and with Michael's support, I sought out Peter one evening during a meeting at Falmouth and made him an offer for the boat in which he had taken the title. 'Sorry,' was his reply, 'I sold it just this afternoon.'

Nothing daunted, the next morning we got in touch with Phantom boats of Sittingbourne, and within next to no time we had committed ourselves to buying a 25-foot Phantom which would cost £6,500 for the hull alone. By the time she was fitted out with a floor and seats, two engines and a pair of fuel tanks, gauges, instruments and so forth the bill would be over £25,000. The shopping list just went on and on.

Apart from dashing from one end of the country to the other to be on the offshore racing scene, we moved from Priors Ford to the house in which Michael had lived with his wife in Ashtead, and I took on half the mortgage. Priors Ford was at that time still owned by Tonia, and it was good to be somewhere which I could begin to turn into a home of my own again. I am a very houseproud woman, and I very soon stamped my style on the kitchen, bathroom and our bedroom, and hung a wonderful painting of the original Bluebird in the lounge as well as displaying some of the trophies which Father and Grandfather had won and photographs which I have of them. Most important of all my two dogs, Susie and Smartie, began to make the place their own. They were miniature dachshunds, which I had had for fifteen years. In personality they were very different. Smartie was wrongly named because she did not have an awful lot of brains, but Susie was as cunning as a cartload of monkeys. She knew my every mood – she knew whether I was happy or sad, and if I wanted to cry I could go and cry with Susie and she would lick up my tears. They took to Michael very well, and though he had not had much to do with dogs before he became a real fool with them.

Smartie and Susie had been with me ever since my days with Clifford and so had shared a lot of anguish and change with me. I bought Susie from a breeder in Hampshire. She was just a tiny dappled puppy then and had such an appealing look in her eyes that I could not resist her. I treated her like a baby in those first few weeks that she was with me: I carried her round the house wrapped in a towel as I did my housework, and at night I even woke up at intervals to take her outside to pee on the lawn. Smartie came some months later, and the pair of them kept me going when at times I might otherwise have wanted to give in. They also livened up the later years of Lisa's life, though I suspect she found their puppyish ways irritating at times! Sadly, all three of my precious dogs are no more, but I shall always be grateful that they gave me more than I could ever give them.

The painful truth which now came home to us was

that if our ambitions were to be realised we needed money – much more money than we could muster – to pay for the boat and finance our racing programme.

Already Michael and I had taken out a second mortgage on our house and sold a Jensen which I had. From then on it was a hard slog. We had a book which lists every company in Britain employing more than 200 people, and from this we selected the ones we thought most likely to be interested in sponsoring us. I telephoned each in turn, but in the end had to resort to a circular letter to go with each brochure and I remember sitting up in bed and signing 200 of these letters in one day. Michael took them off to the letter box and we waited.

Two days later there was a phone call from number sixty-nine on the list – the British arm of the Belgian reprographic company, Agfa-Gevaert. Other tentative responses came from Bluebird Toffees in Switzerland, from Campbell's soups, and from a firm run by my uncle, Spectra Automotive products.

Neither Michael nor I had ever been involved in the kind of negotiations we now began. Agfa-Gevaert seemed to be the best prospect and so we arranged to go and see them. We were not sure whether we should go as beggars looking for a hand-out or a confident pair who were offering the company the privilege of sharing in our success. I think we took a midway position, but when we looked at Agfa's representatives across the table they looked and sounded more like enemies than would-be friends. My heart sank when Bob Dickenson, who was then their managing director, almost barked at me, 'Why should we support you?' It was a tough encounter, and we came away exhausted and with no idea whether we had been beating our heads against a wall or discovering a gold mine.

Difficulty in sleeping is not normally one of my problems but that night I tossed and turned knowing that if Agfa gave us their support they would be hard masters, and if they did not we might have to face ten, twenty, thirty or more such interrogations before we got anywhere. 'How will we pay for the boat we've ordered?' I asked myself again and again, and, 'Where is the money coming from to cover the cost of taking part in the events to which we are already committed in the coming season?' All that was without considering our increased mortgage. Our total resources were our day to day earnings in our respective jobs. Agfa – or someone else – held the purse strings, and if those strings were not untied we should have to give up the idea of racing and look rather foolish.

True to their word, Afga rang at noon the following day. The response was more generous than we had hoped for. They said they were prepared to put approximately £55,000 into our first year of racing which included £15,000 towards the boat, the cost of a full programme of racing at coastal resorts around the country and the very considerable expense of taking part in the Round Britain Powerboat Race in July. As an afterthought, Tony Burton, who was to handle the sponsorship for the company, asked whether he and a colleague could see the boat as they knew nothing about racing or powerboat technology but they had at least to be sure that the craft they were financing existed!

It was too good to be true and, though Agfa never had second thoughts about their commitment, I could not get the deal signed and settled soon enough. There was, I think, more than a little Campbell cunning about the way I made sure it was all tied up quickly.

Michael and I were invited to appear with our new boat and to talk about our plans on the television programme *Pebble Mill at One*. This was a live magazine programme broadcast at lunchtime each day from the BBC studios in Birmingham. I took it upon myself to tell Agfa that if they signed the agreement in time their name would be on the boat when she was shown on television. They liked the idea and put pen to paper without hesitation. The signwriter was hard put to it to complete his part of the job in time, and, in fact, the paint was still wet when we set off for Birmingham.

Looking back, I think we were probably foolish to have accepted the invitation to appear on *Pebble Mill at One* as all our plans could have gone so horrendously wrong but, as it worked out, it was a landmark in my life and my racing career. The angle which the programme editor stressed was that I, as daughter of Donald Campbell and granddaughter of Sir Malcolm Campbell, Britain's greatest heroes of speed, was about to launch myself into the racing and record breaking business. At that stage it was all bravado as far as I was concerned as I had no achievement to show in powerboating. To say that this was a landmark may sound like an exaggeration but, for me, that day was the first time I felt that I could be someone in my own right and need no longer be overshadowed by Daddy's reputation.

Our appearance on *Pebble Mill at One* was also a landmark in publicity terms. When *Agfa Bluebird* was launched, a week or two later, on 19 March 1984, every national newspaper from *The Times* to the *Star* carried a photo and cover story. I was interviewed on both breakfast time television channels, in *South East at Six*, on *Woman's Hour* on Radio Four, Gloria Hunniford's show on Radio Two, and for the *Outlook* programme on the BBC World Service. The British Forces Broadcasting Service even invited me to be their guest of the day as a reminder that the Campbell spirit was still a potent force. Agfa had value for their sponsorship money in the first twenty-four hours and within the next six months had attracted publicity valued in the advertising business at five million pounds.

All this was fine for me, but I had sympathy for the powerboat drivers who had been taking part for season after season, who had so much more experience, and many of whom had won trophies and championships,

who suddenly found that the public spotlight had bee
focused on a novice in their sport just because of he
family background. It must have been intensely annoy
ing.

Michael had similar feelings. To begin with he wa
very pleased to be associated with the Campbell her
itage, but he found the connection more and mor
difficult to live with once the media got hold of it
He is all man and was upset that so much of th
publicity centred on me most of the time. He use
to say that he did not like to be in my shadow, an
did not enjoy frequently having to take second place
I was very conscious of this throughout the time tha
we were racing together and made a point of neve
saying 'I' but always 'we'. And that was absolutel
honest, as I could never have achieved anything i
powerboat racing without his tenacity and hard work
I understood how he felt as a man, and it took him
little while to recognise that there were benefits whicl
came his way because media attention was on me.

Two people who heard some of the broadcasts an
read the newspaper stories were Mick and Debbie Gi
dler, who lived not far from us in Leatherhead. Thei
involvement was to become vital to us. As a boy, Mic
had lived close to Daddy and Tonia in Leatherhead, an
Dad had been his hero. His chance to meet Dad cam
when floodwater washed a canoe belonging to hin
down river and Mick recovered it and returned it to him
As a result he became Dad's odd job boy at weekend
and proudly told us that he had just occasionally bee
allowed to sit in *Bluebird*!

When my father made that remark about engineer
he was in no way minimising their importance, an
neither am I. They are wizards who work miracles, an
the more I race the more I recognise how dependent
am on them. Our chief engineer was Doug Ashley fron
whom I had bought my ski-boat. He was interested i
the possibilities I had in mind as soon as we met, an

222

it was natural when Michael and I had turned those possibilities into plans that we should turn to him for help. *Agfa Bluebird* was taken straight from the builders to his garage in Barnet to be fitted out. Just as Leo Villa, Daddy's engineer, had the backing of his wife Joan, so Doug was supported by his wife Marge. Powerboat racing is so time-consuming that if married couples are not in it together it will soon come between them.

Our television appearances and the newspaper coverage had been very helpful, but they also had their by-products. Even before we had taken part in a race I was being invited to speak at lunches and dinners, and charities seemed to believe that it was my vocation in life to open garden parties and bazaars. I did not, and still don't, mind doing any of these things but just before my inaugural season in racing I decided that there were more important things I had to do.

There was the day when a police patrol car stopped me for speeding on the A35, near Dorchester, in Dorset. The policeman treated me to the usual homily about driving too fast and breaking the law, booked me, and then asked if I would give him my autograph for his son. I had to laugh at the cheek of it! It was also ironical that Malcolm had been before the magistrates for speeding on a bicycle when he was a boy and here was I being rebuked in much the same way when I was learning to drive a powerboat.

With a powerboat it is not really so much learning to drive as getting a feel for an experience. You have to remember that the surface over which you are travelling is uneven, moving liquid which is subject to tides and currents. You also have to take into account the effect the direction and strength of the wind will have on your boat. When it is pushed hard a powerboat is flying so comparisons with sailing or motoring can be very misleading. It is a question of sensing the balance of the boat, and reading the wind and water conditions, but however good you are, you know that at any moment a rogue wave can upset anything which you are doing. Good driving has to be instinctive, and when accidents occur it is almost always because of a loss of concentration, or indecision.

I could feel my self-confidence increasing as our weeks of training went by but my sense of Dad's presence was no less. Sometimes it was when I was pushing myself to dare to do something which I had not done before; sometimes it was in a moment of private self-searching. It was not in any way morbid, but more as though all the pieces of a jigsaw had been scattered on the floor and he was helping me to fit them together. I find that even now I want to do things in ways which I think he would approve of, and if I am at home alone and there is a noise in another room my first thought is that it's Dad doing something when rationally I know that it is almost certainly the cat. I do not believe in spiritual presences as he did, but I have a sense that he is there to protect me when I need him.

I took up racing in part to prove myself and rescue myself from isolation. Also I wanted to keep faith with my family's past attainments and take that tradition into a new generation. But even as I came out of the tunnel of grief and uncertainty I could not escape from Daddy's influence.

14

Powerboat racing is quite different from driving on water which Grandfather and Daddy did. To reach the highest possible speed they needed a surface like glass, with scarcely a ripple. Their *Bluebird*s would have moved across the water without any vibration apart from the engine, and the only indication which they would have had that they were moving would have been the sight of what they were passing on the bank – if they ever had time to look. Powerboats run in choppy or rough seas, with waves sometimes as much as twenty feet high, and all the time you are being thrown about. You are aware of movement in every direction, and, at the end of the race, have the aches and pains to show for it. It's like driving a Formula One car, but the track doesn't keep still! While what I do is within the family tradition, I doubt whether either my father or grandfather would have wanted to take part. Similarly, I know full well that there is no way in which I could drive the *Bluebird*s which they did.

In Britain, the powerboat racing season is from May until September, and most events take place in southern England. Boats of varying sizes are classified differently but all compete together over an eighty-five to ninety-mile circuit. This makes the start very impressive to watch but terrifying to take part in. I remember one race from London to Calais and back when we started in the Thames Estuary on the Greenwich meridian. There was room comfortably for about twenty-five boats on the line, but there were fifty-five of us so there was a lot of pushing and shoving to get the best position. In most races you have to navigate your way around a series of buoys, some of which will be several miles from the coast, but however carefully you have worked on your navigational plan you cannot know in advance where the very sizeable items of junk will be which are afloat in the sea and which can badly damage a boat at high speed. In the river Thames you will encounter a selection of shopping trolleys, railway sleepers, beer kegs and the like any day that you drive.

Competitive sports have to be divided into those which depend solely on your own physical effort, technique and tenacity, and the ones in which a boat or some other machine is involved. Powerboating is obviously in the second category and anyone who takes part has to recognise that however much skill and guts you have the machine can always let you down. You also have to remember that a powerboat allows nothing for comfort or convenience. Both driver and navigator, and the third crew member in the larger boats, are in metal racing type seats so cannot move during a race. Food and drink are impossibilities, first because there would be nowhere to put them but more because to remove your helmet, which would be necessary if you were going to take refreshment, is a sign that you are withdrawing from the race. It is man and woman against the elements with little or no help unless things go wrong. There is radio contact with the shore, but only for use in emergencies.

Buying and maintaining a boat is a very expensive business, and if you have not got the resources to finance an adequate back-up team you may as well not start thinking about offshore racing. On the other hand, there are very wealthy competitors who will have a fifty-strong support group working with them. When I was at the World Championships in Florida, in the autumn of 1987, the owner of the Popeye's Fried Chicken chain in the United States was there with three boats in the Super Class and a back-up team which had at their disposal a helicopter, a fixed wing aircraft and motor scooters. All his helpers were in designer gear in the company colours. Add to that the cost of tow trucks, hotel accommodation, fuel, mechanics, hospitality, and travel from one venue to the next, and you are talking in mega-bucks. And even then he did not win.

It is not surprising that when Michael and I first appeared on the scene the long-established teams did not take us seriously. Our first race is one we shall always remember. It was the Spithead Trophy at Portsmouth in May 1984. Conditions were just about ideal and we were second across the line, but as we were the first mono-hull to finish we could say that we won our class. It seemed that powerboat racing was a piece of cake. That impression was put right at Fowey, in Cornwall, two weeks later. The sea was so rough that the marshal stopped the race halfway through. *Agfa Bluebird* was banging and bumping as she flew off the top of one wave and then hit another. It seemed impossible that she could survive in one piece or that we would have any engines on the stern when we finished. To our amazement, we had covered most of the circuit when the race was called off and we were the winners.

Happily, our best day ever was one when our sponsors had invited 350 guests. We won our class, and took prizes for the fastest lap, first woman and best-presented boat, and even so we had been unable to find one of the marker buoys. We slowed down to look for it and spotted a fellow in a boat pointing to his deck. There was the buoy – well and truly punctured. The rest of the pack caught us when we reduced speed and we had a fight to get away from them again, and it all added to the sense of achievement at the end of the day.

Slowly Michael and I were accepted in the power-boating fraternity, and I think we proved ourselves when we won both the Championship of the UK Off Shore Boating Association and the National Championships of the Royal Yachting Association in our first

season in 1984, and then went on to the European i[n]
1985. It sounds smug, but when other people in the spor[t]
began to measure their performances by ours I though[t]
we had arrived! 'We were second to *Agfa Bluebird*' wa[s]
praise indeed.

I find it impossible to be balanced about our achieve[-]
ments. I get a hell of a kick out of driving and lov[e]
winning so there is the danger that I overestimate wha[t]
we have achieved. The fact is that there are lots o[f]
people around the world who have done much bette[r]
than I have, and have sustained that standard over [a]
number of years. Even at my best, I know that I hav[e]
done only what plenty of other drivers could do – an[d]
that is proved to me almost every time the flag drops fo[r]
the start of a race. Much as I enjoy winning, I also enjoy
other people's success. Their attainment is a challeng[e]
to me, and I know I could do much better than I hav[e]
done. I have very good loyal supporters in Agfa, bu[t]
their commitment is not enough to provide the back-u[p]
to make me world champion.

Given the choice, I always prefer to drive rather tha[n]
navigate, but running as a team I know that the role[s]
have to be swopped from one race to another. In th[e]
larger boats and in very heavy seas a woman can fin[d]
herself at a disadvantage as a driver from the point o[f]
view of physical strength. I also have to admit that I a[m]
not as good as I ought to be at coming from behind, a[s]
I get demoralised too easily, but put me in front and I'l[l]
stay there.

Before a race I always take *Agfa Bluebird* out half a[n]
hour before the start to get my bearings. Then I switch off
the engines and relax while other competitors come ou[t]
in their own time. With five minutes to go a flare signals
that you should go into the muster area and move roun[d]
in an anticlockwise direction. You will already have bee[n]
told on which side of the start boat you should be, so
you move forward, jostling for position with no quarter
given at speeds of 40–50 mph – perhaps sixty abreast

228

– and when the officer of the day drops the Union Jack away you go at full throttle. At that moment you are so close together that you could shake hands with your neighbour. If you are the number two in your boat in a particular race, before the start you are saying, 'Steady . . . steady . . . faster . . . steady,' and then when the flag goes you scream, 'Go!' All the boats are on the move before the start, but as all those engines open up to full power when the flag drops the noise in unbelievable. I love it. For onlookers, that is probably the best part of a powerboat race to watch.

Throughout the race, number two, who is the navigator, has the chart and gives directions to the driver. You will have been given details of the laps which make up the circuit about a week in advance, and will have worked out the compass bearings and hazards to avoid at home before the race day. So it's, 'You're on a good course . . . head for that point to starboard . . . See that buoy in the distance? That's where we turn . . . See that ferry just gone through? Watch for the wash . . . You'll hit his wash n-o-w.' It is so noisy that all communication between the two of you is by intercom, and if that fails the driver can feel very lost and alone.

When you are driving all your attention must be on the water ahead of you and coping with waves and currents. All the information from the gauges has to be relayed to you by your number two. I maintain that the shortest way between two points is always the quickest, and know that very often I have moved up a place in the field by slowing a little and doing a turn very close to a buoy rather than taking a wide sweep as some of my fellow-drivers do. I go into a turn as fast as possible, then drop the boat into the water to reduce speed, quickly change course, and accelerate away.

In the number two position you have the compass between your knees and the tossing about which you get ensures that you have some very tender leg muscles the day following the race. You also need to keep an eye on the amount of water coming into the boat, and often will need to switch on the bilge pumps.

We always split powerboating into three percentages: 50 per cent is your engineer because if the boat breaks down you are not going to get anywhere, 30 per cent is the navigator, and 20 per cent the driver.

At the end of it all I almost dread getting out of the boat. You take your helmet off and your hair is a tangled mess because of the salt water and sweat. You look slightly like a punk as the white of the salt is on your eyebrows and lashes. If you have been driving your hands will be sore, and sometimes my bum has been red raw as a result of the bouncing which you get all the time. During the race you can feel the water creeping down the back of your neck which makes your race suit adhere to your skin, which is very uncomfortable. If the weather is rough, I really dread the race in the hour or so before it starts and I am always slightly frightened. It is a sport in which you can get seriously hurt, and there is the saying, which echoes in my mind, 'The sea takes no prisoners.' It is one of the sad ironies of life that you could be killed doing something which is so exhilarating. I do not have to race and I would not do it if I did not enjoy it, but I still admit to fear and grumble about the discomfort. I know that if I have several months without racing I miss it, and when we are about to set off again the smell of the fuel and the noise of the engines excite an orgasm, the physical stimulus is so great.

In terms of achievement, I suppose Michael and I reached our high spot with the Round Britain Race in 1984. It was the first time the event had been staged for seventeen years, and it involved driving the 2,000 miles or so around the coast of the British Isles in a clockwise direction. We decided at a fairly early stage that it was enough to prove that we had the logistical skill and stamina to complete the course without bothering too much whether we were first or last. Everyone stopped at the same pre-arranged places, but between ports of call we scarcely saw any of our rivals.

With that perversity which makes summer in Britain full of surprises, we set off from Portsmouth on a July day with a force seven gale in prospect. I think the organisers allowed the event to go ahead as Prince Michael of Kent was there to start us, but they were taking a great and unnecessary risk in such conditions. Of forty boats which set out only fifteen reached the first day's destination, which was Falmouth.

After fighting our way through the most enormous seas I have ever encountered between the Isle of Wight and Portland Bill with only one engine working, we pulled into a sailing club at Weymouth. It was quite clear that we were not going to be able to get the faulty one working, so we had to find a truck and trailer to take *Agfa Bluebird* to Falmouth, where our support crew were expecting us.

Our instructions included emergency telephone numbers to be used in circumstances such as ours, so that a search for us did not begin. The response I got was a recorded message inviting me to leave my dinner order after the bleep. I wanted to say that I'd have spaghetti bolognaise at three in the morning as it seemed that it would be that time before we got there.

From the Yellow Pages I found a man in Weymouth who advertised trailer hire who said, 'Yes, I've got the trailer, missie, that'll sort you out.' A very scruffy looking but most obliging young man in a clapped-out Ford Capri joined us before long. His trailer would have taken a sixteen footer without any trouble, but *Bluebird* was twenty-five feet. Nothing daunted, after a bit of discussion and head scratching, he said that he had noticed that a much larger trailer had been chained to a post at a roadside not far away for a couple of weeks. Without more ado, he went off with his wirecutters to collect it, saying that he was sure that whoever owned it would not mind if we 'borrowed' it. To make a comic situation complete he chained his much smaller trailer to the post in place of the one we were going to use. Michael and I, still novices in this game, felt rather embarrassed arriving in Falmouth with our boat on a trailer. We need not have worried. Lady Arran, the doyen of powerboat racing in Britain, had to have hers brought in on the back of a fish lorry.

Race rules said that if you failed to complete a leg as long as you made an effort you could continue, though the number of penalty points set against you made sure that you would not win.

Next day we had to round Land's End and get to Fishguard, in South Wales. I have never been as frightened as I was while we were going round Land's End, and hope never to be again. We realised how foolish we had been to attempt this race in a twenty-five footer, when other people were using forty-six foot boats. There was a thirty-foot sea running and all we could do was to climb up one side of a wave and surf down the other. If you have been to Land's End you will know that it is all rocks with no beach, so there was no question of landing. I said to Mike, 'Oh hell . . . I wanna go home,' and I looked behind us and it was more terrifying than looking straight ahead. I have never felt more helpless. We were near enough to see the coastguards at their lookout but they never saw us and did not log us as having passed them as we were so often in the troughs of the waves. We could not even switch off the engines and wait for things to get better. We were taking water over the top all the time which soon upset the electrics and everything: switches, steering wheel, and gear lever were all live. We knew there were two possibilities – we were going to make it, or we were not. It was as scaring as that.

By the time we were off Newquay we were in real trouble. We had shipped a lot of water and because of the electrical problems the bilge pumps were not working so we had to pull in.

Mike and I must have looked a funny sight plodding up Newquay High Street in our wetsuits, thoroughly dishevelled, dripping a trail of water behind us. All we had with us was my Access card. Suddenly I had hysterics. Mike said, 'What the hell are you laughing at?' His socks were slowly changing from white to yellow. On the way round Land's End he had said over the intercom, 'God, I want a pee,' but, of course, there was nowhere to stop. Some minutes later I heard him go, 'Ooh.' I said. 'What are you doing?' 'I've just peed,' he said. And that's the way it has to be in a race like the Round Britain. You just pee in your suit. Walking through Newquay the pee had run down his legs and was saturating his socks.

We went into a department store not only looking scruffy, but smelling repulsive too. We selected T-shirts, jeans, shaving gear, some shampoo and a couple of cans of drink and then went into the fitting rooms to take off our racing gear and put on dry clothes. We followed our wet footprints out of the shop with our wetsuits in plastic bags.

For the night we found bed and breakfast accommodation and before we went to find something to eat I washed out Mike's socks and put them with his shoes to dry on the radiator in the television room. When we came back after the meal, our hostess said that she did not understand why no one was watching television that evening. When I went into the television room I soon knew why: Mike's socks and shoes were emitting a decidedly manly aroma!

After Fishguard our course took us to the Isle of Man, on to Oban, and through the Caledonian Canal to Inverness. The schedule allowed us a two-day stopover in Inverness to lick our wounds and attend to any problems with the boats. Because it is so far north, summer evenings in Inverness are very long and almost all of us in the race got together for an impromptu barbecue. It was not the success we had hoped for as one of the

233

men who said that he knew where to get the very best Aberdeen Angus steaks and to whom we all gave money to buy them was somehow diverted to a pub. We waited and waited, and when eventually he came back he had just one or two rather average looking steaks and a stomach full of beer. I should think he had drunk all the Tartan in town.

The trials of our journey up the west coast stood us in good stead for the homeward trip from Inverness. We went through gale-force conditions again off Fraserburgh and Peterhead but this time with a competence born of tribulation. But there was nothing that could have prepared me for breaking a bone in my foot, and having to spend the rest of the race taking painkillers and with my foot wrapped in six-inch thick foam rubber. Approaching the place at which we had to sign in at Dundee, I put my foot out to stop us colliding with a tug and it was smashed between the two vessels.

Whitby, in Yorkshire, I decided, is the fish and chip capital of the world. Whether it was the fresh air and exercise which had made me hungry I do not know, but I have never eaten such delicious fish and chips as we had there. We were hugging the coast south of Whitby, but after a few days of racing you are not as observant as you should be and we were not sure of our position. We spotted a couple of men in a boat casting their fishing lines so we pulled up behind them, and I called, 'Excuse me. Can you tell us where we are, please?' We must have approached them more quietly than we realised, and the two of them jumped as though they had seen a ghost. What they saw may well have seemed even stranger – a flashy race boat in smart colours decked with race numbers and Union Jacks, and a couple of southerners in posh wetsuits and bright scarlet helmets. One of them recovered himself enough to say, 'Scarborough, luv.' We thanked them and went on our way, just as though we had paused on a country road to ask directions, and they, thinking no more of it, continued fishing.

Passing Spurn Head, at the mouth of the Humber, Michael needed to go to the loo. I suggested that we stop and he could pee over the side, but, to my amusement, he refused to do so in case the men in the lightship were watching. The lightship was about five miles away, so I told him, 'Michael, you may be well endowed, but I am sure that with the best pair of binoculars in the world they're not going to see you.' Toilet arrangements seemed to be a recurring problem on this trip.

One of the oddest experiences of travelling down the east coast of England was crossing the Wash. It is a large inlet of the North Sea which bites into the land, and as you approach it from the north if you are going to follow the coastline you have, as it were, to head out to sea away from the land and forty miles or so later you will pick up the coast again on the other side. It is a test of faith as well as navigational expertise. By the time we got back to Portsmouth we were exhausted but proud.

I was reminded of the danger we had been in on the Round Britain Race when Didier Peroni had his accident in 1987. Didier had been one of France's leading Formula One racing drivers until a crash forced him to retire in the early eighties. He turned to powerboating with great success, and I met him when I was asked to act as interpreter when he was getting a rap over the knuckles for speeding in the harbour at Cowes a year or two ago. After the official left he thanked me for my help in charming English! In a 1987 race he was driving a very unconventional boat which had the deck and hull moulded into one in an almost cylindrical shape, and we chatted before we went to the start. Off the Isle of Wight he hit the wash of a tanker. A wash has three 'humps', and Didier's boat took off from the first, apparently, flew over the second, but hit the third as it was coming down, turned over and continued driving itself into the water at 80 mph. His injuries were not serious but he was drowned. Because of the damage to his legs and thighs in the car crash which forced his retirement, he had an

235

additional harness in his seat and escape was out of the question. The other two members of the crew were also killed in what was the worse powerboat accident ever. What fools we are! That had happened to Didier and his colleagues in favourable conditions, and Michael and I had risked our necks around Land's End just for the hell of it.

During the last race of the 1987 English season a big wave came over the top of us, smashed the visor of my helmet into my face and broke my nose. When I got out of the boat I knew that was the end of racing for me. I was sore, bruised and stiff next day, but, even then, was beginning to say to myself, 'Well, it wasn't so bad after all.' You develop a love-hate relationship with powerboat racing.

The sport is at its best in Italy and the United States, but New Zealand has the most fantastic coastal water and inland lakes to offer for racing. And the forthright do-or-die attitude of their competitors is something I admire. Mike and I first went to New Zealand for Christmas 1984. Dorothy, Daddy's second wife, had invited us to go and see her and her family there. We were given the warmest welcome you could ever imagine, and the children of her second marriage – Max, Lisa and David – treat me now as though I were their sister. Sadly, Dorothy's husband, Hans Wenk, with whom she had many happy years, has since died.

Dorothy told Mike and me that we would be most likely to meet people with powerboating interests at Takapuna, just outside Auckland. A couple of men were there tinkering with their boat and, after watching from a distance for a while, we went along and introduced ourselves. They were as friendly as people in New Zealand always seem to be, and over the next few days took us out in their boat to see many of the islands along the coast.

They also arranged a lunch so that we could meet some of the people who run powerboating there, and out of that has grown a series of contacts which I treasure very highly. I drove with John Garrity of New Zealand in the World Championships which were held there in 1986, and during that visit also took Barry Thompson's place with Glenn Urquhart in one or two races. Barry and Glenn won the previous World Championship in Guernsey, but on the second day in New Zealand had a fearful crash, and Barry was almost killed. While he was still recovering in hospital, there was a race at Lake Taupo – a freshwater lake in the centre of North Island – in which they had intended to take part. Glenn was hesitant as he had so nearly seen his partner killed, yet wanted to find the guts to have a go again. I think I forced the issue by saying that I would race with him. Only later did I discover that the race was on 4 January 1986 – twenty years to the day after Daddy was killed at Coniston.

Just before the race I had a phone call from Daphne, my mother, to tell me that a radio documentary on Dad in Britain had suggested that he killed himself deliberately, and various papers were wanting to contact me for comment. I told the ones who managed to get hold of me that I thought the idea was absolute bunkum. The way in which the media, in Britain in particular, put someone on a pedestal only to knock them down and try to destroy them later is disgraceful. If there was any evidence that my father committed suicide it would be painful enough to me, but there is not, and I find such speculation after all he achieved hurtful to me and boring for other people.

With such thoughts in my mind, and knowing that the boat I would be co-driving had sunk in Lake Taupo on its previous outing and been in an accident in Auckland before that, I gave Mr Woppit a very special hug and kiss before tying him to the steering column. Mr Woppit had gone to Tonia after Dad's death, but, for some reason, when she was selling their former home in Leatherhead she gave him to me and has, I think, regretted it ever since. After he had appeared with me on television, she wrote saying that she had not given him to me 'to make money and publicity out of'. If she cannot understand I feel sorry for her.

My anxiety was unnecessary and the race was an anticlimax. We had to withdraw because the foot throttle fell to pieces. I had similar apprehension before another race in which I partnered Glenn, at Taranaki. There was a very strong wind and a twenty-foot sea so the organisers reduced the course to twelve fairly short laps. Glenn looked at the conditions and said, 'I'm not taking any chances. I don't want to smash the boat up.' I was relieved and took him to mean that we would do a lap and then retire. We did well on our opening lap, largely because I got my compass bearings right, and, whereas other folk missed a couple of buoys, we did the full revised course. As we were leading, Glenn was not giving up. I thought, 'Oh hell, another eleven laps of this.' I was right, and we went on being bounced and buffeted but still keeping the lead.

No more than a couple of miles from the finish, another competitor edged up alongside us. Above, there was a helicopter taking photographs. Glenn, whose first reaction to the conditions had been so cautious, now had fire in his eyes, and was not going to surrender to this fellow who was creeping up on us. Then, everything went blank. The next I knew, I was facing the back of the boat, waist deep in water, trying to stand up on a floor which was as slippery as ice, and someone was peering through my visor. We had come off the top of a wave, shot up into the air and, so other people told us afterwards, lingered there for a second before crashing back onto our side, continuing to go ahead but underwater with full power still on. I had been knocked out, and a para-medic had jumped from the helicopter and was looking into my eyes to assess my injuries. I was fine, but sick to death that we had hit a rogue wave so close to the end of the race.

238

My visits to New Zealand have given me the chance to make many friendships there. Graham Pike, one of the two men whom Michael and I had met working on their boat at Takapuna and who were our first contacts in New Zealand powerboating, came to drive with me in England during the 1987 season. Graham is totally dedicated to the sport and I have the greatest admiration for his professionalism and his ability to handle boats.

The previous year Michael Standring and I had drifted apart. It is not easy to share the tension of a sport such as powerboat racing, and also be at one in domestic arrangements too. Some of the strains of the cockpit had begun to be evident in the kitchen, and Michael's affections turned elsewhere. I cannot pretend that it was anything other than a shattering experience, and it took me a long time to get my life onto an even keel again. There were days when I could have killed him, and there were days when I knew that if he showed up I would want to be in his arms and back in bed again. Michael was not as helpful as he might have been over the material side of the split, but finally it was all sorted out and we can now meet without any feeling of rancour, though we are not likely to race together any more.

My growing contacts with New Zealand and my increasing warmth for New Zealanders led to me becoming part of the only Kiwi team at the World Powerboat Championships at Key West, in Florida, in the autumn of 1987. Everyone there remembered that the previous world champion, the American, Mark Lavin, had been killed at Key West since the last championships when his boat 'submarined' – as we call it – at 100 mph. We wore black armbands as a mark of respect.

At the opening ceremony each team was asked to stand when the name of the country which it came from was called, and their national anthem was played. I was in two minds as, although I had applied for dual nationality, at the time my only passport was British. As I was part of a New Zealand team I stood up with them.

And what a trio we looked. There was Kevin Green, who is well over six feet tall and as skinny as they come, Graham Sutherland, who is square and stocky with the strength of an All Black forward, and diminutive little me. I am a New Zealander by injection, I tell people, and that is good enough for me.

Per capita, New Zealand has more than her share of the world's greatest sportsmen and women, and the national teams excel in international competition at rugby, squash, yachting, powerboating, cricket and tennis. Such success is based on a more universal involvement in sport than I have found anywhere else. In both Auckland and Wellington I have seen people in their hundreds coming out of offices in the evening and going straight to the boat ramp, the cricket nets or the rugby ground. Then it's quick change from office attire into sporting gear. At lunchtime, the streets are full of joggers, and most health and fitness clubs have full memberships.

Wherever you go in New Zealand you seem to be close to water. You can come out of the ANZ Bank building at Lambton Quay, in the centre of Wellington, walk no more than fifty yards, take your shoes and socks off, climb into your boat and go water-skiing. And that's the city centre! The cities are built on the coastal flatlands, and the ones I have visited all seem to have beautiful high-rise buildings with glass, steel or wooden façades giving an air of affluence, with a backcloth of green mountain slopes rising beyond.

The unfortunate side of lots of water and almost universal involvement in sport is that New Zealand has the highest rate of drownings per capita among the developed countries. New Zealanders are born to sail a yacht or dinghy, ride a surfboard or a canoe, water-ski or fish, or just muck around in the water, and they become careless about the dangers involved. They overload their boats, take too much beer, forget their life-jackets or fail to put them on and the outcome is so often tragedy.

Since the end of 1987 I have been involved in a campaign run by the New Zealand Water Safety Council to increase awareness of such dangers. We have made water safety commercials for radio and television, and I have spoken to countless schools and other community groups. The message I try to put across is think ahead, check the weather before you go out in your boat, take your life-saving equipment and flares with you, and – above all – wear your life-jacket. More than 90 per cent of the people who drown would have survived if they had been wearing a life-jacket. Even a fisherman wearing waders to go into deep water should have one on in case he slips and needs its buoyancy to keep him above the surface should he fall and his boots fill with water. I have had so much pleasure on water and in water that if my name and reputation add more authority to the safety message then I feel that I am making a repayment for some of the enjoyment it has given me.

Concern for safety is an aspect of our family tradition. Daddy was almost a fanatic about it whether we were on a boat, in a car or flying. The only exception which I recall was when we took off in a hurry from Lake Eyre with a storm approaching. He would turn a day out on a boat for pleasure into something like a military operation, but rightly so, I now feel. If you only think of the risks of doing something, you will finish up doing nothing. The secret is to identify the dangers and take precautions, although even then things can go wrong. To face an accident without having prepared yourself is as foolish as wrapping yourself in cotton wool just in case anything should happen.

The Royal Society for the Prevention of Accidents tries to make British people more safety conscious in relation to water. They have an uphill task because we do not have the general involvement in water sports which is taken for granted in New Zealand. The staggering fact is that 75 per cent of the people who drown in Britain never intended to get wet at all. It's not just the people

241

who do ambitious things on water who need to take care, but the ones who seem to be in no danger at all. Fishing from a river bank can be the most placid occupation imaginable, but one foot in the wrong place and it becomes lethal.

The Campbells – one, two and three – each in our own generation have been there to thrill, entertain and inspire, but also to show that respect for danger is part of doing anything in which there are risks.

15

At a given moment on a record breaking run, neither Grandfather, Daddy nor I would have been able to tell you exactly where we were in the measured mile. Setting records is all about training and preparation in advance of the big day, and single-minded concentration on driving skill and speed while you are making the attempt. You may be very lucky and notice when you go past the marker which indicates the beginning of the mile, or you may catch a glimpse of the one at the end of it, but this will be a bonus rather than part of your plan. It is even less likely that you would be aware whether you had done half the course, or a quarter, as you are travelling so fast that your position in relation to the whole is changing second by second.

In just the same way, particularly in this business of speed, we can never be quite sure where we are in relation to the beginning and end of life. When Grandfather saw his *Bluebird* jet boat taken away for modifications to be made, he had no idea that his further plans would never materialise. When Daddy left the Sun Hotel, in Coniston, early that morning in January 1967, he could not have known that he would never return. A few seconds or a few millimetres different, and I would have been killed at Nottingham just after I had set the unofficial World Ladies' Water Speed Record. At any point a life can be summed up with a record of achievements, the debris of our mistakes and failures, and the probings of our dreams. On the measured mile we are ourselves never the surveyors nor the timekeeper for our own run, and our plans and errors are perhaps more valuable to those who follow us than what we achieve.

Since a Campbell tramped the 600 miles from his home in Scotland to London in order to better himself, each generation has passed on experiences, and in some cases wealth, which has shaped the life of the next. From Daddy and Grandfather, and those before them, my greatest inheritance has been an adventurous spirit, a restless determination to win, and an unsatisfiable urge to prove myself worthy of them. Our line of Campbells comes to an end with me, so I feel a responsibility to complete what they began, as well as making my own contribution in the measured mile. In some ways it will be related to speed and safety on land or water, in others to the psychology of motivation, in others to the enjoyment of life.

All three, it seems to me, came together in a venture in which my cousins Malcolm, Peter-John, and Donald were involved some while ago. They had been told that when the Second World War finished, Grandfather had not been able to find some of the silver which he had buried on his property at Tilgate, in Sussex. He had wanted to make sure that it was not stolen if there were an invasion, but after the danger was passed he was able to find only about half of it.

Tilgate is now public property, and visitors are not allowed to go to the small island in one of the lakes on which Grandfather hid his treasure. My cousins and a couple of friends dressed up in combat gear one night, blacked their faces and put on masks with the intention of getting to the island. It is no more than twenty-five or thirty feet from the bank and the water is not deep, but it is very muddy and the bottom consists of slippery clay. To add to their difficulties they had only one pair of waders – borrowed without his knowledge from my uncle – and their expedition had been preceded by a lively evening at the local pub.

When the first of the group had waded across to the island he had to take off the waders and throw them back to the bank so that number two could cross, and so on. One of them had to bring the metal detector over, carrying it above his head to make sure that it did not get wet, and the others carried spades.

By the time the fourth member of the party was on the island the others were at work. Surprisingly quickly the metal detector gave its bleeping sound and they began to dig. The intense coldness of the night and the dampness of their clothing seemed to matter less as their hopes rose. Their luck was in. Within next to no time they could see silver, and out from the soil they pulled an ashtray which, in the light of their torch, they could see was inscribed with Grandfather's name and had the outline of his Bluebird car embossed on it. Their excited voices betrayed the fact that they were on the island to the warden who was doing his midnight round. 'Oi,' he shouted, 'Come back here, you kids aren't allowed on that island.' An orderly withdrawal took place. Orderly in the sense that they hastily buried the ashtray again so that the warden had no idea what they were up to. It was somewhat undignified, though, as they had to repeat the wader-throwing process in reverse, and one of them fell short of the bank, leaving the fourth member of the expeditionary force to get ashore with one foot and leg unprotected. It was a cold and unsuccessful outing, and in the end they had to explain to Uncle Brian how they had lost one of his prized salmon-fishing waders. They have sworn to go back again, and I have made them promise that I will be included in the raiding party next time.

I am surprised that my father, as far as I know, never tried to find the family treasures which Grandfather buried, but I'm sure he would have approved of that attempt. He was always looking ahead to see around the next corner, or over the next horizon. When he was killed he had plans for a rocket car using hydrogen

245

peroxide as a fuel to break the sound barrier on land at sea level, and from the mock-up which he had made I think it would have been like sitting on top of an intercontinental missile to drive it. There is a similar car in the USA called Vanishing Point for which claims of an acceleration of zero to 200 mph in one second are being made. Its thrust is so powerful that the driver needs a tight cage round his helmet to keep his eyeballs in place and protect his neck and spine.

There is a point in record breaking at which the safe-guards become so dominant that, even if you achieve your end, you feel that so many outside factors have been introduced that they have diminished your part as a human being. Two things add a great deal of interest to racing and record breaking and when you have made all your preparations they can defeat you completely. One is the weather, and the other is that indefinable thing which is best described as your own form. It affects every human activity and has little to do with how you have slept, whether you have been drinking, or what you have had to eat. In powerboating, we have to sign a form to say that we have had no alcohol in the twelve hours before a race. But you still have days when mind and hand and foot do not co-ordinate as they should, and you finish last when you should have won.

My remaining aims in powerboat racing or in record breaking, I have to confess, are vague. Few things would give me greater satisfaction than winning the World Championship, but with my present level of sponsorship that is out of the question because I cannot afford a large enough back-up team. But I am not going to sit on my backside and complain. The most important thing at this stage in my career is not to stagnate. It could be that new opportunities present themselves in speed on water, or I could turn to cars. I have an open mind, but I hope that the era of irrational challenges in my life is not over.

Perhaps my uncertainty springs from the fact that I

have lived the tomboy role which was expected of me, and now it is time for the more feminine side of me to assert itself. My mother and father each had three marriages, and I am the only child of all of them. With two such manly heroes as Daddy and my grandfather before me, it would have been unbearable for another male to have taken up where they left off, though I think my father would have wanted it to be that way. Things worked out to be much better. I have done much that a son would have done, but he would never have had the relationship with Daddy which I had. I was his daughter – tiny, petite, blonde, blue eyed and with all the vanity of a lady. I like to do my make-up carefully and wear pretty clothes, and make myself look as good as I can. Another male Campbell would have been rather a cliché.

While I was growing up I watched Daddy through his marriages and their break-ups, and through the comings and goings of his many girlfriends, and I saw what unhappiness and heartbreak it caused him and them. I knew then that I would be clever enough to avoid all these pitfalls, but I have just repeated the process. He was a sensual, loving man, and if he were alive now he would probably be pursuing women still. I am a chip off the old block. I need male companionship, and if there is a physical attraction I will give everything to create a full and satisfying relationship. If I am let down, so be it. I look forward to the next one, and keep striving until I reach Utopia – if ever. In a way, I hope I don't because the quest for it is such fun.

My relationship with my father did not really have very much warmth or depth until I was in my teens. Sadly, it ended before it was fully developed, and I wish now more than ever before that he had allowed me to be closer to him when I was really young.

Although my parents separated, I am grateful for my childhood. Of course, I wish my mother had been around, what child wouldn't? What I missed taught me how to respond to less than ideal situations, and has helped me to stand on my own feet now. Anything which makes children sort things out for themselves is often regarded as a disadvantage. Whether experiences have an adverse affect on us is largely governed by how we react to them. I think I turned my isolation in my childhood to my own benefit.

One of the chief benefits is a measure of adaptability which I believe I have. I can accept whatever circumstances I am in, or whoever I meet. While I was growing up, three women in turn took the role of mother in my life. I liked them all, and mostly got on well with them. Of course, it was in their interest to get on with me from the start, as that helped them to get on with my father.

You could say, in an expression which belongs more to Dad's day than mine, I was 'born with a silver spoon in my mouth'. All the houses in which we lived were impressive, we always had a butler and a cook and other staff, and, as Daddy became more and more successful, we had fast cars, aeroplanes, boats in the Mediterranean and holidays abroad. Despite all this, for as long as I can remember I always made my own bed. But now, much though I enjoy a bit of luxury and comfort, these things are not essential. I have made the house in which Michael and I lived in Surrey, and which is now mine, my own special home and I do not need other material things around me.

In case that sounds complacent, I should perhaps add that such limited fame as has come to me in the last few years means that I am invited to take part in quite a number of interesting and enjoyable events, and this may make it easier for me than for some people to be content with what I have.

An example of this was the BBC television programme *Driving Force* in which I was invited to take part. In teams of two we had to drive vehicles – tanks, fire engines, excavators and so forth – in competition. That day I sat on the back of a motor bike driven by Barry Sheene, and he kept saying, 'Get closer, get closer.' Without any warning he pulled an enormous wheely on me. It was just as well he had told me to hang on tightly.

While I was on one of my trips to New Zealand I was asked whether I would take part in a cool water survival test. I had electrodes attached to my body, even on my boobs. And then, with television cameras watching me, I had to submerge myself in water at ten degrees centigrade, which by anyone's standards is cold rather than cool. What I demonstrated was not the effects of cold water on the body, but the power of mind over matter. I refused to let the water make me shiver, and instead of going up, my heart rate went down. I told the instructor that I just warmed myself up naturally, to which he replied, 'That's what we've always said, Gina. When you fall into cold water, to urinate will help you immensely.' It sounds repulsive but it is true, as the urine warms you up inside your suit and will do you no harm.

I am still naive enough to marvel that so many people want my autograph when I take part in the launch of a product at a show. I sometimes suspect that the marketing people are hidden away around the corner paying people to come and ask me to sign their programme, or something, in order to get a crowd at their stand. One thing which amused me, but I could not understand, was when I was on the Afga-Gevaert stand at a printing trade exhibition at Ashford, in Kent, and a fellow who was introduced to me insisted that I could not be Gina Campbell, and that I was a stand-in hired for the day. I couldn't understand why he thought this, or what good it was doing him to insist on it.

Usually I have *Agfa Bluebird* with me at shows, and any aspiring boat builder who comes along cannot resist telling me how her design could be improved to make her go faster. I listen, and very often learn from someone else's ideas.

I enjoy testing cars, too. I have an affiliation with Renault, and the high spot of my test driving for them was the Alpine. It is a GTI, with a V6 turbo. It is the most horny, sexy car I have ever driven, and the whistle of the turbo coming in really turns me on. They are raced in France, Germany and Italy, and I think it is the most exciting car I know.

The thing which has exhausted me most is the Round London Marathon. It is not the kind of marathon which you tackle on two feet, but with a partner in a dinghy. You collect your inflatable and a 5 hp outboard engine at Putney, and the 100 couples set off at 15-second intervals. The winner is not necessarily the first back to Putney, but the couple whose time is closest to an unstated optimum time worked out by the organisers, less penalty points.

Stage one takes you under Tower Bridge to Limehouse Basin where the Grand Union Canal joins the River Thames. The timing is arranged so that you reach this point at low tide which means sloshing your way across 200 yards of mud before climbing a 30-foot wall, dragging your boat with you. There are some steps at one side, but with 100 pairs wanting to use them all at once, it is a fight to get to them, and another fight again to get back down to collect your outboard motor.

Once you have negotiated the wall, you are faced with a stile, a footbridge and a kissing gate before you can launch your inflatable into the canal. They look to be very lightweight craft but I can assure you that when you are carrying them over obstacles and trying to run as well they almost break off your arms.

The Grand Union Canal loops right round the north side of London, and by the time you reach your overnight stop at Little Venice you will have negotiated thirty locks, hauling your boat round every one of them. You will also have created mayhem as you rush through a fruit and vegetable market in the middle of a Saturday afternoon. I discovered that anyone within ten miles of London who has a dog seems to take it to the tow path alongside this canal to evacuate its bowels daily. The second day takes you to Brentford Lock, where instead of the 30-foot wall to climb, you have to drop 30 feet onto the mud and across to the river before your return to Putney.

This really must be one of Britain's wildest events. It has been run by the London Motor Boat Racing Club for the last ten years with sponsorship from Carlsberg, and as competitors have to sign up sponsors it raises a great deal of money for charity. I find that you cannot respond to every charity appeal so I focus my efforts on the RSPCA, the Injured Jockeys Fund and the Spinal Injuries Association.

In my personal life, I have grown up in the last three years. From the time I was seventeen until then I had either been married or within a live-in relationship all the time, and I had no casual love affairs. There was no third party involved in the break-up of my first marriage: Cliffy and I were the best of friends but the extra dimension which makes a marriage just did not materialise. My second marriage ended because I had entered into an affair with Michael, and I knew that once we had begun to make love there was no going back. I am not a two-timing woman when you are living with someone on a married basis. Once there has been unfaithfulness, although both parties may want to patch things up, there is always the chance that later on there are cross words and one will say to the other, 'You're the one who went off and did this or that, and you were quick enough to drop your knickers.' The hurt is always there, and when there is an argument it is always likely to come to the surface again. I admire people who can push an act of unfaithfulness aside, but I am not like that. I take full responsibility for the ending of my second marriage. It was the result of the weakness of the flesh and the circumstances which arose, and no fault of Philip's whatsoever.

I saw a car sticker which said 'single' and then 'and love it', and between the two there was a heart. That

251

sums it up for me. It was hell for months when Michael and I parted, but I have learned to use my independence and enjoy my freedom. I no longer have to account to anyone for my time, my feelings or my loves, my likes or dislikes, my moods, my temperament, or my money. I am not responsible to anybody. As long as I feel that I am doing the right thing, I only have to justify it to myself.

Don't misunderstand me, I have no wish to spend the rest of my life without a partner but most of the men of my age seem already to be well on their way to being boring old men. Ten years ago all my male contemporaries seemed to be charming and good-looking, now they are overweight, unambitious and middle aged.

Perhaps, in the past, I have fallen in love too easily. But now I find that I am asking myself whether those experiences were love at all. And while I have been alone I have met one or two men with whom things have gone well, and we have enjoyed one another, but it has been for a fleeting time and no commitment has resulted.

A man has to have a whole range of qualities for me to be attracted to him. Eyes are very important and very often tell you more than an individual would want to reveal immediately. In what he is doing, he has to be a complete and utter professional so that he commands my respect, and I want him to have the tenacity to see his task through to the end. He needs to be well mannered enough not to offend me, or cause embarrassment in company. I see no virtue in suffering fools, and I do not tolerate mistakes – one maybe, but only one.

By saying that, I have probably consigned myself to loneliness for my remaining years, but I would rather that than be tied to a wimp. If I meet someone who fits the bill and something bubbles up between us I will carry it through, enjoying every second, and knowing that I am not cheating anyone. Although in powerboating I spend a lot of time with men, I am all woman and have strong sexual feelings.

I may go six months without a sexual relationship because I do not meet anyone who turns me on, but if I do, watch out! I may spot a man out of the corner of my eye and I will watch him and know within ten minutes whether we would go well together. Sometimes I have to stop myself when I am aware I am fancying someone, or I know that before long we will be between the sheets. And I am seldom wrong: if I feel it is going to be good, it is because he has been transmitting similar feelings.

Whereas I am decisive about relationships, I am easily swayed about almost everything else. If I am told that the thing over there is black and I think it is red, I will question my own judgement before I'll challenge what I am told. Such trust of what other people say can lead to painful disappointments but I would rather react spontaneously to another human being than always doubt the other person's integrity. This arises, I expect, from Daddy's strictness about honesty. He would never tell me a lie or a half-truth, and would not tolerate me lying to him, or to anyone else. When he caught me out he thrashed my pants off. I expect this of other people. I have been taken advantage of in business, in sport, in love and just about every other activity of life, but I still believe that scepticism is destructive. Take advantage of me, and I will fight back, and win.

Most of my time is spent rushing from one country to another, from one event to the next. But at heart I am lazy. I have no private income and have to live off what I earn, but I tend to think when I have earned enough to travel that I will spend what is in the bank and start work again when I need more money. I admit that this is no way to become wealthy, but then, if I had the money to buy a Porsche, a larger house, or have a boat on the Mediterranean I would probably think of better ways to use it. My only extravagance, I think, is clothes, and I love buying them and feeling that I have the right thing for every occasion whether it is casual or formal.

Sooner or later I shall have to plan what I am going to do when I give up powerboat racing and all that goes with it. My first thoughts had been of marketing designer-style sport and leisure wear using the Campbell name or the Bluebird logo, but that market seems to be flooded with products using the names of other people in sport. Journalism, public relations work or advertising all have their appeal as they are professions which are not as tightly structured as so many others. And I have had thoughts of launching out in the fashion business in partnership with a friend. My father had strong political ambitions, and I find that I have increasingly vociferous opinions and concerns and, who knows, the doors may yet open for me in that direction.

Two other things about me are, in a way, complementary. I believe that tomorrow is not promised to anyone, and I make it my rule never to leave undone the things which I can do today. I could be talked into driving in this or that championship, and take one chance too many which proves to be the last one. The other thing is that I am really worried about growing old. It would depress me to reach the stage at which my mind makes appointments which my body cannot keep. If someone says, 'Do you want to climb Mount Everest?' I want to say yes without considering whether I am too old, whether I am fit enough, or whether I would die of exhaustion or exposure on the way. I want to keep my options open, and accept any opportunity for adventure which comes my way.

Daddy and Grandfather always hoped that when their time came they would die at the wheel of a car or a boat, and after he had seen Grandfather struggle through his last few days Daddy felt still more intensely that he wanted his life to end while he was doing the thing he loved most. Tragically for the rest of us, but happily for him, that wish was fulfilled. I have no death wish, indeed I want the Bluebird of hope to be there challenging with the promise of a greater happiness than I have yet known in sport and in home life, in Britain or New Zealand, for as long as I am around. If it is not, I have no wish to go on living. I do not feel that I will live to be old, but I hope that to the end of the measured mile there will be adventures and hazards to be wrestled with and overcome.

BOOKS CONSULTED

Donald Campbell *Into the Water Barrier*
Leo Villa *The Record Breaker*
Douglas Young-James *Donald Campbell*
Roma Dulhunty *The Spell of Lake Eyre*
Cyril Posthumus *Land Speed Record*
Richard Hough *Book of the Racing Campbells*

APPENDIX ONE

The Bluebird Cars

My grandfather bought the first car in which he broke the World Land Speed Record in 1923. Its previous owner was Kenelm Lee Guiness who had already set a World Record with it at Brooklands. It had been built a year earlier to a design by Louis Coatalen. It was a Sunbeam with a V12, 18,322 cc Manitou aircraft engine, but despite its 350 hp had drum brakes on the rear wheels only. Grandfather modified the engine and added a streamlined nose and pointed tail before getting his first record at Pendine Sands, in Wales, with a speed of 146.16 mph in 1924.

The first car ever built specifically to break records was the Campbell-Napier Bluebird of 1927. It had a Napier 450 hp broad arrow engine, with three banks of cylinders. The chassis was designed by Amherst Villiers, and the mechanical features by Joseph Maina. It was built partly at the Robin Hood Engineering Works, at Kingston in Surrey, and partly at my grandparents' home at Povey Cross. Its first record was also at Pendine, and was 174.88 mph.

In 1928 a further Campbell-Napier Bluebird also had a broad arrow engine but in this model it was a 900 hp Napier designed for the Schneider Trophy Air Race. The body had a long, low nose and a detachable tail fin with surface radiators on either side of the tail. To streamline it there were fairings fore and aft of the wheels, and there were light discs covering the spokes. The sides of the cockpit were higher than previously to protect Grandfather from the slipstream. Its first record was 206.95 mph at Daytona Beach in Florida in February 1928.

The same engine was used with a more streamlined body in the Campbell-Napier-Arrol Aster Bluebird of 1929. The car was much lower but had a distinctive hump around the cockpit which allowed Grandfather to be seated astride the gearbox. The surface radiators were abandoned. It was used at Verneuk Pan in South Africa in 1929. Although it exceeded the record which stood when Grandfather and the team set out from Britain, it failed to match a higher speed recorded in the USA while they were in South Africa.

In a re-designed version for the 1931 attempts, Reid Railton had an off-set prop shaft and gearbox positioned alongside the driving position which still further improved the streamlining. It had a supercharged 900 hp engine, a new gearbox and larger wheel fairings. Its initial record was 249.09 mph – again at Daytona Beach – but this was increased to 253.9 mph the following year, by which time a new nose cowling had been added.

Rolls Royce were involved for the first time in 1933, with the Campbell-Railton-Rolls Royce car which had a supercharged 2500 hp V12 engine, with two bulges to cover the ranks of cylinders, and an air intake for the supercharger in the nose. As with the previous car, the body was built by Gurney Nuttings. It increased the record to 272.46 mph at Daytona Beach in February 1933.

The final version of Grandfather's Bluebird incorporated the same engine as had been in the 1933 model, with the chassis, front axle, brake drums and shoes from the 1927 car. The body was new with an air intake in the nose which could be closed to reduce wind resistance, a new back axle with twin wheels out of alignment, and double crown wheels and pinions. It was built at Brooklands, and gave Grandfather his last land speed record of 301.13 mph at Bonneville Salt Flats in Utah in 1935.

Daddy's Campbell-Norris-Proteus Bluebird of 1960 had a Bristol Siddeley Proteus free turbine engine which developed 5000 hp. It had four-wheel drive and two gearboxes with a fixed ratio, as the engine had enough power at lower speeds for gear changing to be unnecessary. There were three independent braking systems, and complex electronic instruments. The design was by the Norris brothers, and it was built at Motor Panels Ltd., at Coventry. In the early stages of its trials in Utah it was wrecked, but was rebuilt and a stabilising tail was added. In 1964 it pushed the record up to 403 mph at Lake Eyre in Australia.

APPENDIX TWO

The Bluebird Boats

The *Bluebird* single-step hydroplane of 1937 had a Rolls Royce R-Type 2500 hp engine like the one used in the last pre-war Bluebird car. Designed by F. W. Cooper with Reid Railton as mechanical consultant, it was built by Saunders Roe with a mainly wooden hull and a single screw. At Lake Maggiore it set a record of 126.33 mph, which it later raised to 131 mph at Lake Halwill, both in Switzerland.

In 1939 Reid Railton suggested a three-pointer. A three-pointer planes on two sponsons on the bow and a third is part of the transom. Again it was built mostly of wood, had a single propeller, was designed by Commander du Cane and built at Vospers. Coniston Water was the scene of its first record – 141.7 mph – in 1939.

When record-breaking resumed after the war, the three-pointer was given a Goblin jet engine, and was considerably modified by Vospers. The boat proved to be unstable at speed and was not a success.

After my grandfather's death in 1949, Daddy had the original Rolls Royce R-Type engine installed in *Bluebird* again, and eventually converted into a prop-rider, which means that the propeller became the aft suspension point. In 1951 she hit a log and sank.

My father's success came in a jet *Bluebird* designed in 1955 by the Norris brothers. This *Bluebird* had a Metropolitan Vickers Beryl engine developing 3750 lbs thrust, a metal hull and an off-set rudder. She was built by Salmesbury Engineering. Ten years later Dad had a Bristol Siddeley orpheus engine fitted which had a thrust of 5000 lbs, and it was in this *Bluebird* that he died.

261

APPENDIX THREE

Grandfather's Records

On Land:

September	1924	146.16	Pendine Sands, Wales
July	1925	150.86	Pendine Sands, Wales
February	1927	174.88	Pendine Sands, Wales
February	1928	206.95	Daytona Beach, Florida
February	1931	246.09	Daytona Beach, Florida
February	1932	253.97	Daytona Beach, Florida
February	1933	272.46	Daytona Beach, Florida
February	1935	276.88	Daytona Beach, Florida
September	1935	301.13	Bonneville Salt Flats, Utah

On Water:

September	1937	126.33	Lake Maggiore, Switzerland
September	1937	129.5	Lake Maggiore, Switzerland
July	1938	130.93	Halwill, Switzerland
August	1939	141.74	Coniston Water

APPENDIX FOUR

Father's Records

On Land:

July	1964	403.1	Lake Eyre, Australia

On Water:

July	1955	202.32	Ullswater
November	1955	216.2	Lake Mead, USA
September	1956	225.63	Coniston Water
November	1957	239.07	Coniston Water
November	1958	248.62	Coniston Water
May	1959	260.33	Coniston Water
December	1964	276.3	Lake Dumbleyung, Australia

In 1964 my father became the only person ever to break both world Land and Water Speed Records in one calendar year.

MORE BIOGRAPHIES AVAILABLE FROM
HODDER AND STOUGHTON PAPERBACKS

CHARLES HIGHAM & ROY MOSELEY

☐	35844 0	Cary Grant: The Lonely Heart	£4.99
☐	39250 3	Audrey: A Biography of	
		Audrey Hepburn	£2.50
☐	41122 2	Orson Welles	£3.95

MINTY CLINCH

☐	41200 8	Harrison Ford	£2.95

JOYCE GRENFELL

☐	50238 X	Darling Ma: Letters to her Mother	
		1932–1944	£3.99

JOHN PEARSON

☐	50598 2	The Life of Ian Fleming	£4.50

All these books are available at your local bookshop or newsagent, or can be ordered direct from the publisher. Just tick the titles you want and fill in the form below.

Prices and availability subject to change without notice.

HODDER AND STOUGHTON PAPERBACKS,
P.O. Box 11, Falmouth, Cornwall.

Please send cheque or postal order, and allow the following for postage and packing:

U.K. – 55p for one book, plus 22p for the second book, and 14p for each additional book ordered up to a £1.75 maximum.

B.F.P.O. and Eire – 55p for the first book, plus 22p for the second book, and 14p per copy for the next 7 books, 8p per book thereafter.

OTHER OVERSEAS CUSTOMERS – £1.00 for the first book, plus 25p per copy for each additional book.

Name ....

Address ....

....